M.C

THE
FORGOTTEN HOSPITAL

An Essay

MICHAEL HARMER

Springwood Books

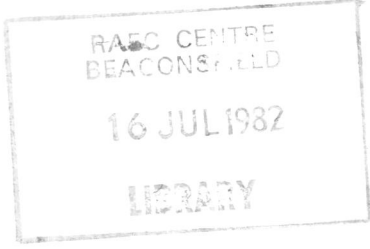
First published in England by
Chichester Press Limited
in association with
Springwood Books
1982

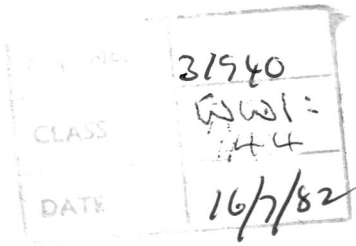
© M. H. HARMER 1982

ISBN 0 86254 100 X

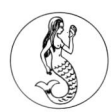

Printed in England by
Chichester Press Limited, Chichester, West Sussex

for

WILLIAM DOUGLAS HARMER

and

THE ANGLO-RUSSIAN HOSPITAL

In piam memoriam

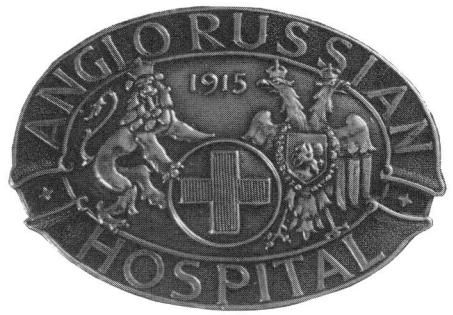

CHAPTERS

APPENDICES

ILLUSTRATIONS

See Notes on the Illustrations, Appendix 5.

Prologue

This Essay was provoked by the finding of 54 letters written by my father from Petrograd to my mother in England, together with a short diary which he kept when he was the senior surgeon to the Anglo-Russian Hospital in 1915-16. At about the same time I also read Mr Wilfrid Blunt's biography of Lady Muriel Paget[1] who was the *fons et origo* of the hospital. It was upon these sources that initially I depended for my narrative and I must say at once that I am most grateful to Mr Blunt for the information which his book provides and for his permission to quote from it so extensively.

When I began writing I soon discovered how very little was known about the hospital. For instance there is no record of its activities, or even of its existence, in the official *Medical History of World War I*. The Royal College of Surgeons and the Royal Society of Medicine could tell me little, nor could the Royal College of Nursing. The British Red Cross Society, through its archivists, generously gave me all the information which was available in their records and were able to provide several documents and facts of importance. Surprisingly perhaps, the definitive history of the British Red Cross Society, written by Dame Beryl Oliver, mentions the hospital in only a single paragraph;[2] an indication, I fear, that it was in fact a very small item in the immense work which the Society undertook during the First World War.

Subsequently, as I began checking references and following leads, I was most fortunate in being able to secure the help of members of the families of Lady Muriel Paget and of Lady Sybil Middleton. This help is acknowledged, I hope appropriately, at the end of this Essay, but at the beginning of it I have to say that without the veritable cornu-copiaeias of letters and documents which they were generous enough

[1] *Lady Muriel.* Wilfrid Blunt. Methuen & Co, London. 1962.
[2] *The British Red Cross in Action.* Beryl Oliver GBE, RRC. Faber & Faber, London. 1966.

1

to put at my disposal my efforts at describing the history of the hospital would have been a poor thing indeed. Inevitably I have a lot to say about Lady Muriel and Lady Sybil and their activities but it is no part of my brief to attempt any sort of assessment of their characters. Should I unwittingly have given offence I would plead, like the Baker in *The Hunting of the Snark:*

> You may charge me with murder — or want of sense —
> (We are all of us weak at times):
> But the slighest approach to a false pretence
> Was never among my crimes!

The Anglo-Russian Hospital, or Hospitals actually, since there was always a base hospital in Petrograd and up to three field hospitals operating in various parts of the Eastern Front, was functioning between its arrival in Russia in November 1915 and its somewhat hurried exit, following the Revolution, in January 1918. It was admirably supported by the British Colony in Petrograd as well as by the Russian Red Cross, and it will be necessary to explain something of the administrative arrangements which kept it going. How it came into being, who staffed it and what it did are told in the course of my narrative, but who were behind it was just as important, and from a biographer's point of view a good deal more interesting.

In brief, the hospital was proposed by the Foreign Office for excellent political reasons: funded by a public subscription, supported by a large donation from the British Red Cross Society and the Order of St John of Jerusalem in England, organised by the sort of people who well knew how to organise such things, and run initially by a small number of dedicated amateurs who knew virtually nothing about such matters at all. The BRCS were in a difficult position. They had been very much involved with the hospitals which had gone to the Balkans in 1912 and 1913 and they had found themselves unable to look after the staffs of these hospitals when they had been over-run or captured by the enemy for the simple reason that they were not official Red Cross hospitals. So while supporting the Anglo-Russian Hospital enthusiastically, the BRCS disclaimed 'ownership' of it. I am obliged to the BRCS for an explanation of this important point. In the Second World War they sensibly imposed a more rigid discipline: either they ran a hospital completely or they left it to others to do so.

In the event therefore the hospital resembled one of those mythical beasts whose front-end consisted of one animal and whose after-end, another. In this case it might be appropriate to suggest an eagle's head and a lion's body if only because the emblem of the hospital, which is reproduced on the title-page and which incidentally was taken from a woodcut made by Lady Muriel's husband Sir Richard Paget, depicts the British lion and the double-headed Russian eagle supporting the Red Cross and the date of foundation of the hospital. It was an enterprise which was intended to be entirely self-supporting, 'a Gift from Britain to Russia'. This is what the original Appeal made clear and the fact that it did not work out that way is no reflection upon those who believed in the ideal. The chairman of the organising committee was himself a high official of the BRCS. The medical staff were chosen on advertisement or on personal recommendation. The nursing staff were similarly engaged, though a considerable number were either Red Cross nurses or VADs. Behind it, the Foreign Office exerted a patrificial presence. It was an enterprise which seemed eminently reasonable in 1915 but I doubt if it would be so considered to-day.

To understand the background it is necessary to recall something of the situation on the Eastern Front during the 18 months following the outbreak of war on 4th August 1914. And in particular perhaps to learn the names and situations of the various places which will be mentioned. To take countries first. Poland and Finland as we know them to-day were Russian; that is to say they had been provinces of Russia for the previous 100 years. The same was true of the Baltic States which had curious names like Kurland, Livonia and Ingria; and of the border areas between Russia and the Austro-Hungarian Empire, Galicia and Bessarabia, which latter country formed the left bank of the Danube at its outlet to the Black Sea.

Then there were regions, roughly designated (as for instance, East Anglia or the Midlands) such as Volhynia and Podolia: and to make confusion worse confounded, Lithuania was an immense area which had once stretched from the Baltic to the Black Sea but was now more usually known as West Russia. At all events it was over this territory, which included the dreadful Pripet Marshes, that most of the fighting occurred and where the field hospitals were engaged. Next, the towns themselves kept changing their names. St Petersburg became Petrograd in 1914 and of course eventually Leningrad: Helsingfors in Finland was renamed Helsinki after that country achieved its independence. Worst of all were the Baltic towns which, according to whether they were German or Polish or Russian, had a bewildering variety of names. Fortunately few of them require identification in this narrative, and those that do, although possessing tongue-twisting names like Voropayevo, Molodechno and Rozhishche, will be found on to-day's maps if anyone cares to look for them. It may be appropriate to add a note, if only in self-defence, about the spelling of Russian names. When quoting extracts from letters and despatches I have left things as they were written (even when they were clearly incorrect); but I have tried to record them, in my own text, in accordance with present usage. The termination -ff therefore becomes -v, as in Kiev (for Kieff) or Ignatiev (for Ignatieff). The reader will doubtless find many other apparent inconsistencies.

It is also necessary to summarise briefly and of course quite inadequately, the broad outline of the campaign which raged between Russia and the Central Powers, Germany and Austria, from the outbreak of what the Russians now call the 'Imperialistic War' until the Revolution in 1917 and the Treaty of Brest Litovsk in March 1918, which ended the war with Germany as far as Russia was concerned.

On the outset of hostilities, the Central Powers attacked across what is now Poland and rapidly over-ran that country, including Warsaw itself. The Russians, for their part, struck back in the north and south. Their invasion of East Prussia was a total failure and they lost 150,000 prisoners alone. To the south, in Galicia, they advanced far into Austrian territory and would have swept on had it not been for the entry into the war of Turkey, on Germany's side. This opened up a new frontier in the Caucasus and it also closed the Straits, making it impossible for supplies and reinforcements to reach Russia through the Black Sea. The failure of the Allies at Gallipoli and Salonika to re-open this route compounded the disaster.

The following Spring the Germans advanced *en masse* across Poland and by May 1915 the Russians had lost over one million men. Moreover they had been pushed back in the south as well, in bloody fighting which led, as I shall explain, to the reason for the establishment of the Anglo-Russian Hospital. The year 1916, which is for the most part the one covered in this narrative, went somewhat better on the Eastern Front. General A. A. Brusilov, who had shown much promise as a more junior commander in 1914, was given control of a new offensive in Galicia and which was launched on 4th June 1916. By the end of this campaign he had taken over 400,000 Austrian prisoners but the losses in dead and wounded were colossal. It is in this theatre that we will find the A-R Mobile Column in action.

4

Meantime in Petrograd the government were becoming less and less able to keep charge of affairs at home or at the front. The Tsar himself assumed the rôle of Commander-in-Chief and appointed ministers, often on the advice of the Tsarina and the scheming 'monk' Rasputin, who were incapable of controlling events. The political system of Russia has been described as Absolutism tempered by Assassination and at this time the seeds of revolution, which had been sown in 1912, were germinating, and as everyone knows they flowered in 1917 first in Petrograd and later all over the country.

If my father is the hero of my tale, my heroines are Lady Muriel Paget and Lady Sybil Grey, the co-directors of the hospital. Had I to choose between them, I think that Lady Sybil Grey would come in first by a short head; but it would be a close-run thing. Lady Muriel was the entrepreneur, the true organising genius; Lady Sybil, the administrator. Together they made a splendid team. Throughout my narrative I refer to these two ladies in this fashion and to my father as WDH, except in that chapter which describes his letters to my mother where I use a more personal style for each of them.

I have adopted the device of adding footnotes as I go along, and this idea I borrowed unashamedly from Gibbon, who used them to such good effect in his *Decline and Fall;* and perhaps for the same reason, that they may enliven a somewhat dull account of what was nevertheless an interesting and unusual experience.

In 1965 I visited the Soviet Union, in the main to inspect their three finest cancer hospitals and in order to meet some of their distinguished oncological specialists. Fifty years is a considerable time of course but I was both surprised and disappointed to find that not a single doctor I talked to had even heard of the existence of the Anglo-Russian Hospital. One of these was Prof. A. I. Rakov, the Director of the Leningrad Oncological Institute, who I knew well. Following his death I wrote to his son, a haematologist in Leningrad, asking him if he could give me any information about the hospital and explaining that it had been established in the Dmitri Palace. He replied: 'I have managed to find information that such a hospital really did exist. It was located on Nevsky Prospekt, House no. 41.' *Sic transit gloria mundi!*

On my return I wrote a brief account of my visit. I called it *Behind the Arras* and I subtitled it with Hamlet's farewell words to Polonius, words which may be considered equally suitable in regard to this Essay: *Thou wretched, rash, intruding fool...*

WDH

When my father volunteered to join the staff of the Anglo-Russian Hospital in 1915 he was 42 years of age. It may be wondered why he did so. He had been appointed to the staff of St Bartholomew's Hospital as a general surgeon in 1903 at the unusually early age of 30, an indication of his brilliance in this field. He was already Warden of the Medical College, a post which was traditionally held by a bachelor. He lived in the hospital in a nice house overlooking the Square, surrounded by the four splendid Gibbs' buildings (which recalled the more famous one at his own college at Cambridge) and which centred upon the Fountain, the symbol of the hospital.

As Warden he was responsible for the welfare of all the students, pre-clinical and clinical; their selection, their studies, their examinations, their successes and their short-comings, which were in those days considerable. It involved an immense amount of work and which today is organised by a dozen or more people. He dealt with all correspondence himself, having been refused the services of a part-time secretary by the Medical College. The Warden whom he replaced had been both lax and ill, and there was an immense backlog of work to be coped with (he found a drawer of letters, many of which were unopened and some of which contained cheques for students' fees which had never been cashed) and so he engaged a secretary at his own expense. In addition he was the emergency surgeon to the hospital and this entailed many long hours of operating during the night watches.

His predecessor had actually died of galloping consumption while in office and in residence: and so, in view of the infectious nature of tuberculosis and the strain under which WDH was working at the time, it is little wonder that he too developed the disease. In fact this did not become evident until after his marriage in 1906. It is difficult to imagine a more disastrous start to married life. Leaving the Warden's House at St Bartholomew's, he and my mother moved to 45 Weymouth Street, on the fringes of the more distinguished Harley Street, where they established their home and in which he had his

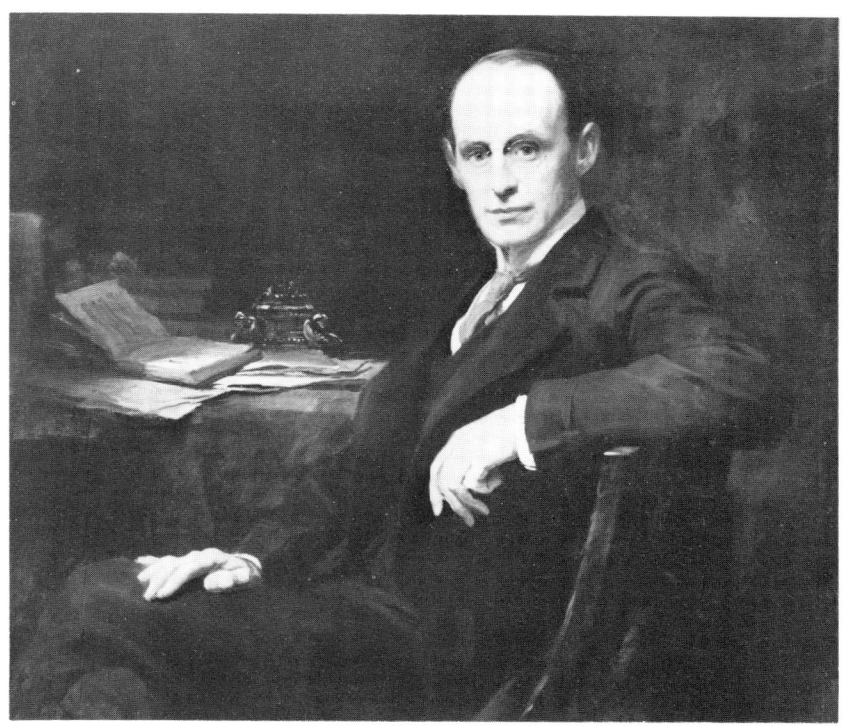

WILLIAM DOUGLAS HARMER

consulting rooms. Within the year he developed pneumonia 'which did not resolve' and his colleague Dr John Drysdale, who had been best man at his wedding and who was acknowledged to be the best chest physician at Bart's, diagnosed miliary tuberculosis, then (as even today) a mortal condition. In retrospect this must have been an error — there was little diagnostic radiology at the time — but clearly the disease must have been extensive and it was certainly deemed to be of a most serious nature.

He was advised to go to Switzerland 'for the cure' and at Davos Dr Huggard told him that he would recover and lead a normal life. The prospect of a year in a sanatorium was not altogether displeasing because he was an ardent skier, having learned the art in Norway, and indeed he was one of the first ever to take skis to Switzerland and elsewhere. At the Annual Dinner of the Ski Club of Great Britain in 1908 a tour through the mountains of Montenegro was proposed 'to ascertain whether there were suitable slopes and snow for ski-ing'. In spite of the annexation of Bosnia and Herzegovina by Austria it was decided to go ahead and WDH, with three others, left Arosa in Switzerland in January 1909 for an expedition which lasted a couple of weeks. His experiences were described in the *St Bartholomew's Hospital Journal* the following November. The 'madness of the Englishmen' was suspected as being a cover for subversive activities and they were quite lucky not to be incarcerated. It was at Davos in February 1907, in the midst of a monumental snowstorm, that his first son and my eldest brother Richard was born. WDH returned to England 'cured' and in fact he was cured because he never showed any further evidence of this lung affection during the 88 years of his life. However, at the time it was argued and he was advised, that the life of a general surgeon would be too demanding and in consequence he was persuaded to take charge of the newly formed Throat Department at St Bartholomew's. In the event he worked just as hard in this developing speciality as he would otherwise have done, but I believe that he always regretted leaving the field of general surgery, which was itself at that time beginning rapidly to extend its frontiers. He was fortunate to have had the advantage of being trained by the best surgeons of the day during a decade when it had been conclusively demonstrated that the principles of antisepsis could be improved upon by the practise of asepsis in the operating theatre. As a student he had seen the bloodstained frock-coat (which it was said was capable of standing up on its own) in use: and although that was a thing of the past, the new-fangled rubber gloves were still something of a joke and the healing of operation wounds 'by first intention' was by no means usual.

WDH was a bold and technically advanced operator. For instance, he was one of the first to divide the sternum or breastbone, in order to operate within the chest. He saved the life of a young meat-porter from Smithfield Market, whose liver had been ruptured in an accident, by finding the tear and successfully suturing it. Thirty-two years later, when I was a house-surgeon at Bart's, I was examining a patient who was to undergo an operation the following day. I noticed a huge scar in his upper abdomen and enquired as to its nature. He replied that he had torn his liver in an accident in the Market and had been admitted more or less dead. A surgeon sewed him up he said, and then he added; 'and funnily enough, he looked rather like you'. I went to the basement record store and in piles of dust located his notes. It is a fact that I bore a striking resemblance to my father but it also illustrates the astonishing retrieval power of human memory. WDH had a critical mind concerning contemporary opinion and convictions of his own so it is not surprising that he did not take too kindly to the thought that he was being pushed into the 'backwater of Throats'.

When war was declared in 1914 St Bartholomew's Hospital undertook the responsibility of staffing, with doctors, nurses and auxilliaries the First London General Hospital in order to cope with the casualties from the Western Front. Here WDH was able to revert to the rôle of general surgeon. There was at that time no conscription but many doctors were volunteering for service, which in the main meant the Army. He already had the honorary rank of Captain RAMC at the hospital but his health record precluded active service in France. I believe myself that it was his wish to serve actively which led him to volunteer for the staff of the hospital unit which was despatched to Russia in late October 1915. The Anglo-Russian Hospital Committee had recently been established in London and the newly appointed Commandant now wrote to WDH in his own hand:

Dear Mr. Harmer

I am writing to tell you that Mr. Waterhouse is going out as Senior Surgeon and that we will not have a vacancy for another Senior Surgeon at present. I am sorry you are not coming with us, but at the same time I doubt your being altogether strong enough to stand a severe winter should we be subjected to much hardships.

I have been asked to suggest a good operating surgeon to go out to Cannes as Second-in-Command of the South African Ambulance there. It is an institution of 200 beds. Would you care to go? I believe it carries the rank of Major RAMC.

This letter is undated but clearly WDH did not care to go because before long another letter from the Honorary Secretary of the Committee arrived. This time it carried a date:

Dear Sir   November 16 1915.

It has now been decided that you should leave England to take up your duties in the Hospital at Petrograd on Wednesday next the 24th inst, travelling by the 2.20 pm from Kings Cross on that day and proceeding from Newcastle to Bergen and then overland to Petrograd.

Perhaps if WDH had taken the post at Cannes he would have

escaped developing the middle-ear infection, during the severe winter to which they were indeed subjected and which eventually necessitated a radical mastoid operation. Ironically too, a few days before he was due to leave he was offered the post of Commandant of an Advanced Base Hospital at Le Touquet. Having accepted the Russian assignment he turned this down and his place was taken by his friend and colleague at Bart's, Charles Gordon Watson. I do not know if he regretted his decision though I think that my mother may have done. For his work at Le Touquet, in which he certainly did sterling work, Gordon Watson received a KBE. My father may also have missed the accolade on a second occasion when he operated upon the Prime Minister, Mr Bonar Law in 1923. He had been called in by Dr Gould May (of whom we will hear more in this account) and Sir Thomas (later Lord) Horder, who considered that the P.M. might be suffering from cancer of the larynx, on which disease WDH was certainly one of the best opinions in Britain. An exploratory operation, done in conditions of some secrecy in Mr Bonar Law's house, failed to provide a definite diagnosis. The P.M. was grateful and asked Horder: 'Do you think I should recommend Harmer for a Knighthood?' 'Harmer wouldn't be interested in that sort of thing', he replied. 'Perhaps not', my mother is said to have remarked, 'but his wife might have been'.

My father never talked much about his time in Russia, apart from some personal anecdotes, but his letters and diary leave little doubt that it was a disappointment to him, at any rate in terms of useful surgery and compared with what was happening in Flanders during 1916 where the flower of British surgery was engaged in almost ceaseless work. He was actually with the hospital for a comparatively short time, 11½ months to be exact though in fact this was a longer period than all but two of the other doctors. The normal tour-of-duty was six months before home leave, but he did not return to England when he might have done because there was at the time no one to replace him. It is interesting to speculate whether he might have gone back for a second tour. As I shall tell later, he was pressed to do so and indeed it seems to have been assumed that he would do so. But he clearly missed his family tremendously, he was anxious about his professional future and there were financial considerations to be taken into account. So in the event he did not go back and as far as I am aware, never expressed any wish to visit the USSR. In this he differed totally from Lady Muriel Paget who adored Russia and to whom I now turn my attention.

Three Ladies

During the Second World War the *Aid to Russia Fund,* under the chairmanship of Mrs Winston Churchill, raised seven and a half million pounds. Mr Churchill himself wrote: 'My wife felt very deeply that our inability to give Russia any military help disturbed and distressed the nation increasingly as the months went by and the German armies surged across the Steppes'. In the First World War there was equal sympathy in Britain and throughout the Empire for the terrible sufferings of the Russian troops on the Eastern Front. Though the sum subscribed between 1915 and 1919 was a mere fraction of that donated between 1941 and 1947 the desire to help and the effort instilled was of the same degree of magnaminity. Moreover the reasoning was very much the same. Mrs Churchill sensed not only the desire to help but also, in the absence of the Second Front for which the Russians had been clamouring from the moment of Hitler's invasion in 1941, the need to demonstrate something practical in the way of aid. As in 1942, so in 1915. The Head of the British Military Mission, Sir John Hanbury-Williams, was importuning the Foreign Office for some 'gesture' in lieu of the military aid which the Russian leaders demanded and which quite evidently it was not within the power of the British and the French to provide.

This gesture was supplied during the early summer of 1915 by a quite remarkable woman who 'saw suddenly where her destiny would lead her'. Muriel Finch-Hatton[1] was the daughter of the 12th Earl of

[1] Subsequently Lady Muriel Paget. Born 1876, died 1938 aged 62. Lady Muriel Paget CBE has to be distinguished from another dedicated Red Cross worker, Leila Lady Paget GBE who was the wife of the diplomat, Sir Ralph Paget KCMG. In 1912 and 1913, when he was British Minister to Serbia, she had organised hospitals during the Balkan wars. From November 1914 to February 1916 she established and maintained 'Lady Paget's Hospital' at Uskub (now Skopolje) on behalf of the Serbian Relief Fund Committee. During the frightful typhus epidemic, when smallpox, diphtheria and scarlet fever were also rife, her hospital 'became an inferno of infectious diseases' *(BRCS Joint War Committee Reports).* Lady Paget herself contracted typhus and nearly died from it. For her services she was awarded the Order of Saint Sava, 1st class, the only uncrowned woman ever to be so honoured. A description of Lady Paget's Hospital is given in *The Quality of Mercy,* by Monica Krippner (David and Charles, 1980).

Winchilsea. According to her mother, who insisted on the truth of it, she spoke her first words at the age of three when she said: 'How pretty the garden looks today, Mamma' — a nice fragment of family lore.

She had been brought up in the aristocratic milieu of those times and at the age of twenty-one had married Richard Arthur Surtees Paget, a young barrister known to his family and friends as Artie and to his colleagues as RASP. In 1908 he succeeded to the Baronetcy of his father and in due course became a brilliant scientist-inventor. Referring to his achievements in later years, Sir George Thomson FRS wrote this: '. . . a grand representative of the class of men who love science for its own sake and are amateurs in the finest sense, holding no office and looking for no reward: would that there were more of them now!'

An engaging story, which I remember hearing as a boy, may well be current to-day; that he dreamed up the astonishing idea of training sealions to detect German submarines. In fact he was a pioneer in the investigation of soundwaves transmitted through liquids and which in due course led to the development of Asdic in all its forms. It was Sir Richard who coined the word supersonic (so well known to-day) but which he later changed to the more accurate term ultrasonic, by definition sound waves having a frequency above the range of the human ear. In connexion with this story Blunt has a delightful account, in his biography of Lady Muriel, of the occasion when 'in the chilly waters of the Westminster Swimming Baths, from which the public had been rigorously excluded, the First Sea Lord and several high officials of the Admiralty watched suspiciously as the choicest of the performing sealions stared at the water with distaste but was finally persuaded into the bath, where it performed to perfection in homing-in to the appropriate sound'. Sir Richard also later immersed himself in the Firth of Forth and, having perfect pitch, recorded the note which had been transmitted from a distant microphone with exactitude. If he were able to read that the mating call of a whale may now be detected 3,000 miles away in the Pacific Ocean I feel certain that he would be the first to admit humility: but the point of the story should be that, as Secretary to the Submarine and Electrical Section of the Board of Invention and Research of the Admiralty, he was actually training Admirals and not only sealions.

In spite of indifferent health and many infirmities throughout her life, not least the one that ended it, Lady Muriel fought against them

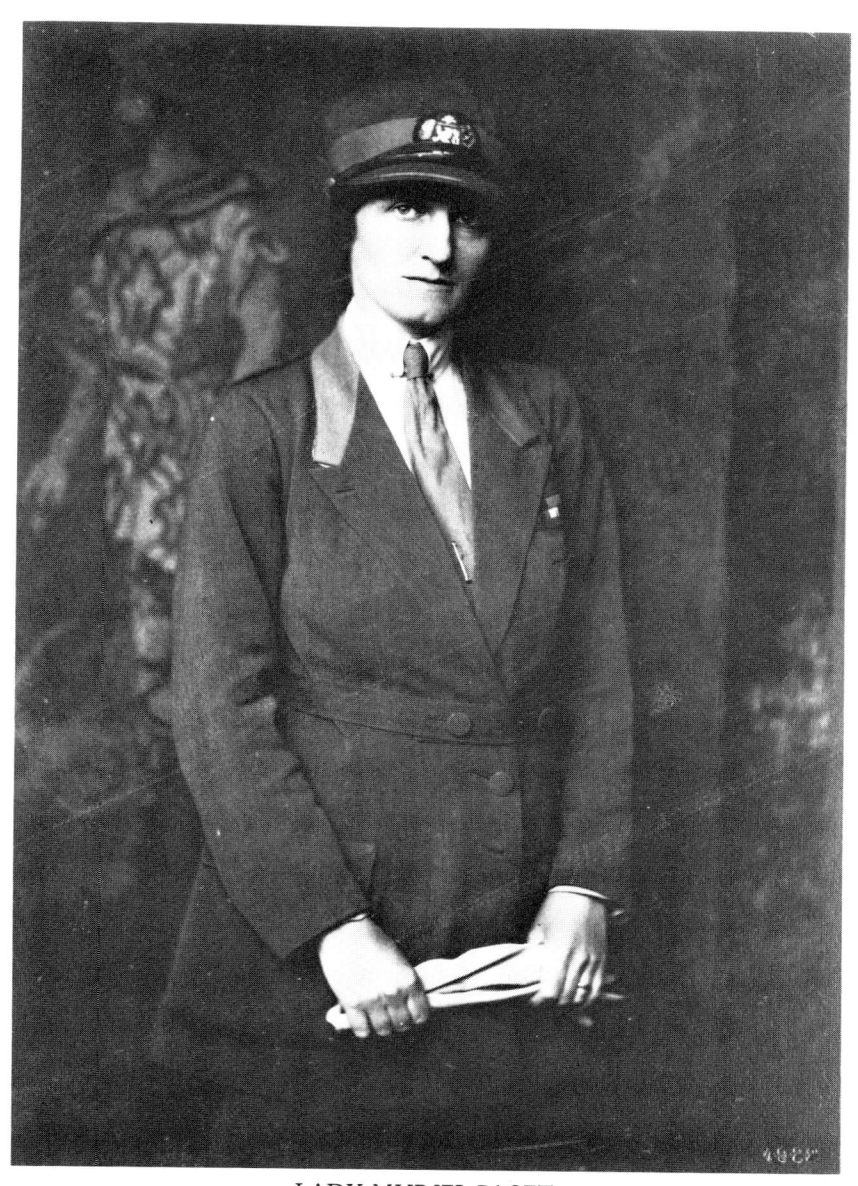

LADY MURIEL PAGET

all with tremendous courage and determination. It is said that when her time was running out she answered the customary polite enquiry with the reply: 'Very well thank you, except for a touch of cancer'; and that at a time when this was almost an unmentionable disease.

When the A-R H. was running out of steam in 1918 her restless energy took her off to Slovakia in answer to a plea from her friend Alice Mazaryk that the plight of the returning refugees in the aftermath of the war was desperate. She had been asked to organise a new hospital in South Russia at the same time but preferred Slovakia.

When officials criticised her lack of plans she was wont to reply in one of her favourite phrases — 'Rubbish! Don't be so fussy!' She went to Versailles where the Allied statesmen were remaking the map of Europe to seek support for her efforts and Dr Beneš, the newly appointed Czechoslovakian Foreign Minister, who had other matters as well to consider at that time, is reported to have remarked: 'Protégez-moi, protégez-moi de cette dame!'

After Slovakia, the Crimea, Latvia and then back to Russia itself where she embraced the cause of the Distressed British Subjects — the D.B.S. — 'because nobody else was willing to do so'. Little wonder that her youngest daughter, when asked by a school friend what it was like to have a mother who was always in Russia, replied that, 'to me a mother *is* someone who is always in Russia'.

These anecdotes have little to do with the Anglo-Russian Hospital it is true, but they may serve to indicate what a very remarkable couple I am attempting to portray.

To return. Lady Muriel's adored younger brother had died in 1892 when he was only nine years old from one of those so-called inter-current infections which would be regarded as quite trivial to-day: and six years later she was to suffer the double agony of losing her own first born son, Richard, at the age of six months fron infantile gastro-enteritis. The year before his death, her brother had, as a tutor, a young man called Bernard Pares[2] and he had persuaded Muriel to join 'a society interested in Russia'. This was actually The Anglo-Russian Committee of which Pares was the Secretary from 1909 until 1914. Now, 24 years later he met her again, having recently returned from Galicia where he had been with a Red Cross unit attached to the

[2] Subsequently Sir Bernard Pares KBE, he became Professor of Russian History and Literature at Liverpool University and a general authority on all matters Russian. His book *My Russian Memoirs* (Jonathan Cape 1931) includes a fascinating account of the year 1916 with which this Essay is mainly concerned.

Russian 3rd Army. He was able to speak with authority, having witnessed the appalling sufferings of the peasant-soldiers as they retreated before the Germans during the winter of 1914. He told her of the terrible shortage of munitions, of the vast number of casualties, of the need for field hospitals and medical equipment. Above all he spoke of the heroism of the Russian soldiers. Pares spent most of the war years in and out of Russia collecting information for the Foreign Office and acting as the official representative of the War Office with the Russian armies on the Eastern Front. We shall meet him again in this account.

Others were saying the same at this time. There was for instance Hugh Walpole, the novelist, who served with an *otriad* during the retreat of 1914-15 and who wrote:

> The magnificence of the Russian soldier is surely beyond all praise. I wonder if people in France and England realise that for the last three months here he has been fighting with one bullet against ten. He stands in his trench practically unarmed against an enemy whose resources seem endless — but nothing can turn him back — whatever advances the Germans may make I see Russia returning again and again. I do from the bottom of my soul, and what is of more importance, from the sober witness of my eyes, here believe that nothing can stop the impetus born of her new spirit. This war is the beginning of a world history for her.

We shall meet Walpole again too; and also a Miss Florence Farmborough. She had gone to Moscow in 1908 to teach English to the two daughters of a Russian heart specialist, Dr Pavel Usov, and to learn the language herself. In 1914, having enlisted with the Russian Red Cross, she too witnessed that winter's retreat in Galicia. Throughout the war she kept a diary which remained unknown (except to her family) until it was published many years later.[3] In her book there is a most moving account of the wounded which it is appropriate to quote at this point:

> The patience, the sustained endurance of the heavily-wounded is heart-rending. If anyone should ask me what I consider the outstanding qualities of the Russian soldier, I would have no

---

[3] *Nurse at the Russian Front. A Diary 1914-1918.* Florence Farmborough FRGS (Constable, London 1974). Miss Farmborough was 86 at the time of publication and died in 1978.

hesitation in replying: patience and endurance. Sometimes as I watch them lying there on their beds of straw, so still and composed, despite the pain which their wounds must be causing them, I try to imagine what they must be thinking . . .

A nurse's feelings perhaps. A surgeon's might be expected to be more prosaic so to complete the quartet I now add WDH's recorded opinion:

The Russian soldier is an ideal patient. His powers of resistance are indeed marvellous. Practically every patient who came under our care was a countryman, accustomed to live in the open air, inured to extremes of heat and cold and able to undergo major operations with a minimum of shock.

At the age of 39 Lady Muriel 'determined that she should do something about it and the idea of forming a unit of English surgeons and nurses as a gesture of good-will occurred to her'. It may not have been quite as simple as that but there is certainly no doubt that it was due to her energy and devotion that the Anglo-Russian Hospital came into being. Pares disclaims, or at least does not mention, any influence which he may have had in this connexion and in fact his *Memoirs* only contain the briefest of references to the hospital. It appears possible that it was Earl Grey who persuaded the Foreign Office to set up a Committee. At any rate this was speedily done under the Presidency of Lord Cromer and with Major-General Lord Cheylesmore KCVO as Chairman of the Executive Committee and Lady Muriel herself as the honorary organising secretary.[4] Queen Alexandra, whose sister was the mother of Tsar Nicholas II, accepted the Patronage.

The organisation of the unit went well. Staff were enlisted, equipment purchased and that vital necessity shipping, arranged. An Appeal was launched by the British Ambassador in Petrograd who emphasised in a letter to *The Times* on 30th August 1915 that 'The Russian Red Cross warmly welcomes the proposal and authorises me to say that it is not so much money, but a Hospital, equipped and staffed, that it needs at the present moment'. Two weeks later the same newspaper

[4] The full Committee is given in Appendix 2. Considering that the A-R H. was really a trivial item when set against the whole content of the war effort it is a matter for astonishment that it numbered no less than 108 members. It would be fascinating to know how many times it met and what the quorum was! Apart from Queen Alexandra, it included both Archbishops, the Prime Minister, several members of the Cabinet, two Field Marshalls, Earls, Lords and Lord Mayors. It also included Sir Starr Jameson, Lady Muriel's 'Beloved Doctor', after whom she named her son, the present Baronet, Sir John Starr Paget.

16

published, as was customary, a whole page advertisement of the first list of subscriptions. It was headed by His Majesty the King (£100), Her Majesty the Queen (£50) and Her Majesty Queen Alexandra (£100). There were three subscriptions of £1000 and the Russian and English Bank of Petrograd donated 10,000 roubles (at 20 to the £). There were a few in the hundreds with a fair sprinkling of guineas, but for the most part they were in double or single figures. It had been announced that to equip a unit of 200 beds for one year would probably cost £30,000.

The first list raised £13,299 5s. 4d., so although a start had been made the Committee had much to worry about. A brochure was published from which it may be seen that some hard work must have gone on behind the scenes. 'The Dominion of Canada has sent a splendid contribution of £10,000' — Earl Grey's influence, I do not doubt. 'The employees of the Elswick Ordnance Works have voted a sum of £500' (an offshoot of Armstrong-Vickers at Scotswood, Newcastle.) 'The Royal Scots Greys, the Regiment of which H.I.M. the Czar is Commander-in-Chief, have presented and provided for the maintenance of five beds'. The idea of endowing beds caught on and all over the country towns and districts began doing so and in due course would have the fact recorded in English and Russian on an appropriate plaque above each bed. The Royal Automobile Association presented four ambulances and some private donors did the same. Thirty individual firms gave equipment and the list makes fascinating reading, ranging from linen, dressings, bandages and so on to Bovril, Jeyes' Fluid, Thermogene Wool — and champagne. They ran into a spot of trouble here, as did the Red Cross itself. Their *Joint War Committee Reports* for 1915 suggest an agonising situation: 'The department received large quantities of wine, champagne, port and sherry and it was decided to distribute it to hospitals during Christmas time. The experiment was not repeated . . . a distribution of this character involved an infringement of the Defence of the Realm Act, under which no patient in hospital could be given alcohol without a medical prescription.' Even Gibbon might have found himself at a loss to comment appropriately! Contributions continued to arrive. H. Hoskier Esq gave a mezzotint of Miss Campbell by Sir Joshua Reynolds, dated December 1778; 'to be sold for the benefit of the Hospital. Offers are invited'. The Scottish Branch of the British Red Cross Society 'moved by a like impulse, has sent £5000'. Soon the Committee were able to announce:

The equipment of the Hospital, including Operating Theatre, X-ray and Bacteriological Outfit, will be complete in every detail and adaptable for field or base work on the lines of communications, according to the final decision of the Russian military authorities.

All was set for departure when, at the last moment, Lady Muriel 'was taken ill with blood poisoning' and a substitute had to be found. It was presumed that this locum would only have to hold the fort for a short time but Lady Muriel 'did not regain her health so quickly'. When I came across that statement it struck me as most improbable that 'blood poisoning' would have kept her — of all people — out of commission for six months (because it was not until the following April that she arrived in Petrograd to assume her duties). Mr Blunt was unable to give me the evidence for this diagnosis, having destroyed the notes from which he had written his biography 20 years before, but both Lady Muriel's daughters agreed with my scepticism and it therefore became necessary to look for other reasons.

There seem to have been four other possibilities.

John Paget had been born prematurely in November of the previous year and had weighed only three pounds at birth. Having lost their first son it is reasonable to suppose that the Pagets would have had grave anxieties about the survival of their second, particularly as he was far from well — 'a touch of pneumonia' (Sir Richard) — during his first year of life. To one who was himself a paediatric surgeon, this seems to me a likely reason. I do not know of course: but there is a second curious explanation which was given by 'L.E.J.' in his obituary of Lady Sybil Middleton many years later.[5] 'On the eve of the departure of the Hospital, its leader, Lady Muriel herself, was found, to the general dismay, to be in what could still be referred to as an interesting condition . . .' I must say that medically this seems to me to fit the facts, but I must also add that there is no other evidence in support. Certainly nothing came of it.

The third possibility is less dramatic and has been suggested to me by Lady Muriel's daughter, Pamela Lady Glenconner. Among the earliest and most abiding of her mother's interests were the 'Invalid Kitchens' which she had set up in the East End of London in 1905. By the Autumn of 1915 the original five centres had increased to 17 in order to cope with the demands of the war; and the organisation of

[5] Her brother-in-law, Sir Lawrence Evelyn Jones Bt. *The Times*. 19th June 1966.

these, 'from Fulham to Finsbury and again from Poplar to Paddington' as a newspaper article remarked, required an immense effort. It is possible that Lady Muriel simply felt that she could not leave England at that time.

Last and certainly probable, is the fact that the London Committee were still much concerned about fund raising. Since Lady Muriel was the organising secretary it may well be that she could not be spared at that time. Had this been so I think there would have been some indication in the records. There is none that I can find: so the problem must remain unsolved.

Lady Sybil Grey[6] took her place. She too was of the aristocracy, the eldest daughter of the 4th Earl Grey, sometime Governor-General of Canada and himself well versed in Anglo-Russian affairs. He was many other things as well. The letters PC GCB GCMG GCVO LLM JP speak of a life in the public service and to these may be added Member of Parliament for South Northumberland and Tyneside for a six-year period before he succeeded to the title. A Whig by upbringing and a Reforming Liberal by inclination, he supported many of the causes which were developing about the turn of the century — Proportional Representation, the Wholesale Co-operative Movement and above all the promotion of Imperial Unity. One of his heroes was Mazzini, the saint of the Italian republican movement and like him he sought to bring men to see political perfection. Another was Cecil Rhodes, whom he regarded as the greatest visionary of his generation. He had many far-reaching ideals, the reform of the National Church being one and he also believed that, given the opportunity, he could have solved the Irish Question. During his last illness he enquired the name of the nurse who had been engaged to look after him and when she replied 'Rainbow', he observed cheerfully, 'I've been chasing rainbows all my life'. He was a most lovable and loving man, seeing good in all and evil in none.[7]

Sybil and her younger sister Evelyn had been with him in Canada between 1904 and 1911 and had shown themselves to be 'the most excellent ADC's'. It is certain that his character affected their outlook on life and inspired them to emulate his achievements. So it is not

[6] Subsequently Lady Sybil Middleton OBE. Born 1882, she died in 1966, in her eighty-fourth year.
[7] See: *Albert, Fourth Earl Grey. A Last Word.* Harold Begbie. (Hodder and Stoughton. 1918.) Born 1851, died 1917.

surprising that, at the age of 33, Lady Sybil accepted the task — a totally unknown task — of establishing a Base Hospital in Petrograd and two or three Field Hospitals at the front, wherever that front might be. It is true that she had been the first VAD to be accepted by the Royal Victoria Hospital in Newcastle upon Tyne when war broke out in 1914 and was not long after appointed Commandant of the Howick Hall Convalescent Home, her parents' Northumberland residence. This hardly fitted her for the direction of a hospital in far-off Russia and the manner of her appointment seems so extraordinary by to-day's standards that it is worth recounting in some detail.

At breakfast one morning in August she simply received a letter from Lady Muriel asking her to take her place: and, as simply, accepted by the afternoon post. The Cheylesmore Committee had unanimously accepted Lady Muriel's recommendation and that was that. (It had in fact been approved by the Foreign Office as well.) At that time few organisers of such enterprises had any of the training which would now be considered mandatory but they had the confidence to embark on them and the determination to carry them through. It cannot be said that her appointment was generally received with approval. A medical journal is on record as describing it as scandalously inept and the *British Journal of Nursing* was in a rare state of indignation:

> The Nursing Profession we think, has a right to know why a young untrained girl is to be placed in this responsible position when a very highly trained and experienced Matron has been selected and a staff of twenty-four certificated nurses have been engaged.
> The reply to this question will no doubt be as usual — that the trained nurses will be in charge of the hospital and that their duties will not clash. Bitter experience proves that it is most difficult to retain discipline under the system of dual control and that when an untrained Lady of Title — backed by social influence — is placed in supreme authority in a military hospital, disorganisation in the Nursing department is inevitable. Let us hope that the Committee will consider this defect in its organisation before it is too late.

One might have supposed that at least Lady Sybil's proud mother would have taken some offence at this tart observation, but not at all. Having been shown the Leader in the *BJN* by a Sister at Alnwick

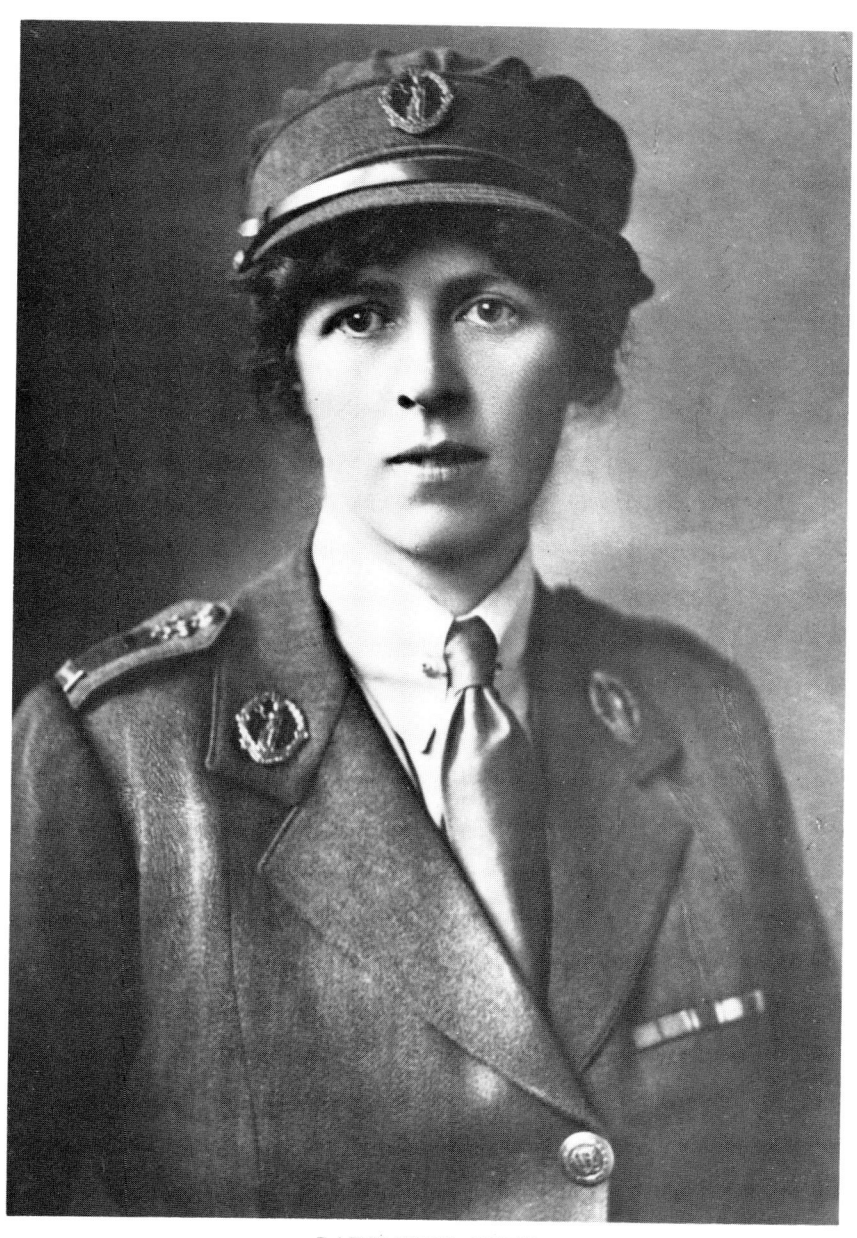

LADY SYBIL GREY

21

Hospital she wrote to her daughter:

> Darling. I shall not write much to-night, as it is already late and I want to go to bed; I am enclosing you a delicious effusion about you and the position you are — usurping. I think the phrase about the Lady of Title etc. should be framed and hung up on the wall of Alnwick Castle Hospital.

'Little did they know', wrote L.E.J. in the obituary to which I have already referred. 'By her coolness, her wisdom, her imperturbable commonsense, her charm, her warm human sympathies and above all, her unselfregarding devotion to duty, Sybil Grey made an outstanding success of her job.' It was indeed not an easy one. She was prepared to give orders to a number of quite distinguished men, some of whom were old enough to be her father; to look after 50 assorted nurses and VAD's and not least perhaps, to satisfy the standards of a very determined Matron. She knew her mind and did not mince her words. 'It is absolutely necessary when you send out fresh men that they should be up to date surgically (she wrote to Lady Muriel). Men like Paget and Williams know *absolutely* nothing about it. They are quite useless'. And again: 'I told him that we have a chance of getting a young and good surgeon who is over in this country and that the opportunity was too good to lose and that he was rather too old for the job'. And on a third occasion: 'There is no doubt Jefferson is a first-class surgeon, especially for a Base. He is a little too slow for the Front'. Well, she was certainly on a winner there. *O tempora mutanter!* Would such a thing be possible to-day?

Because of Lady Muriel's absence, Lady Sybil was in complete charge of the hospital from November 1915 to April 1916. She found the accommodation, organised the alterations and arranged for the arrival of patients; and all this during a winter of almost unparalleled coldness, even by Russian standards. In one of his letters WDH wrote that the lowest temperature they experienced was 67½° below freezing-point Farenheit (minus 37.5° Centigrade) and he added, 'a temperature of this sort does not encourage the Ward Sisters to open the windows'. Nevertheless they insisted on doing so, to the dismay and consternation of their patients! Lady Sybil faced other troubles as well. She had to suppress a near mutiny of the medical and nursing staff who felt that they were wasting their time, was bullied by telegrams from Lady Muriel in London and eventually had to sack the hospital Commandant. Moreover at a critical stage in the hospital's career she had the misfortune to be severely wounded in the face by a fragment of shrapnell and had to return to England for three months.

There is no doubt that Lady Sybil won the admiration of the doctors.

The third lady was of a very different kind. Lady Georgina Buchanan[8] was the wife of the British Ambassador to Russia, a diplomat of the true Establishment. He had been accredited to both Berlin and Vienna before being appointed to St Petersburg at the age of 59: so he knew a great deal about both aspects of the conflict. Of him Pares wrote that '. . . his simple and noble character was proof that we had an altogether exceptional Englishman as the representative of our Sovereign. He had a kind of baffling simplicity . . .' Maybe he did: but it was supported by the traditional British diplomatic guile. The Tsar was in the habit of reading *The Times* with his breakfast and this newspaper usually arrived at the British Embassy in the diplomatic bag on the preceding evening. Sir George would go through the paper and delete any criticisms of Russia, substituting more appropriate paragraphs which were then inserted in identical type, before the paper was delivered to Tsarskoe Selo the following morning. An anonymous English expatriate recorded that 'the Ambassador is adored here and most highly thought of. I don't know what would have happened if there had been a fool or a malingerer in his place'. Geoffrey Jefferson recorded his opinion more briefly: 'Sir George is a rum-looking bird, rather like a stage Englishman in the USA'. Sir George had married in 1885 and so Lady Georgina may have been in her mid-fifties at this time. Blunt describes her as 'stately, formidable, energetic, indiscreet and quick to take offence: a generous friend but a dangerous enemy. She worked indefatigably at her British Colony hospital'. Hugh Walpole, who was by then Chief of Allied Propaganda, was more concise: 'Lady Georgina, *when she likes,* is the kindest person in the world . . .'.

It was 'The British Colony Hospital' which might well have provided the seed of discontent, for this was Lady Georgina's personal baby. Originally established as a convalescent home it was soon enlarged to meet the needs of the war. Janet St Clair put the matter rather more bluntly than one feels was approved by the Embassy at

[8] Born Georgina Muriel Bathurst, daughter of the 6th Earl Bathurst: married the Rt. Hon. Sir George Buchanan PC, GCB, GCMC, GCVO: died 1922 at about 62 years of age.

that time.[9] 'First the management got rid of the officer's wards and sitting room, as the hospital now receives soldiers only; then they turned their *five large committee rooms* [my italics] into a spacious ward.' This decision to take 'other ranks' was clearly a political one and it applied to the Anglo-Russian Hospital also when this was opened. It was a far-sighted decision too because in 1917 when the revolutionary mob several times invaded the A-R H. Lady Sybil was able to persuade them to leave on the grounds that there were no officers among the patients.

The hospital was staffed by both Russians and British. A Doctor Martinoff was the head surgeon and Mrs Froome 'acted as matron' though the senior sister was Russian. To assist there were Miss Tyack, 'a fully trained English nurse' and Miss Field, 'trained for some time in Cambridge Hospital'. It is not my intention to question the abilities of these women nor of Miss St Clair herself who had joined the staff after nursing at Vilna during the first German advance: rather to wonder whether such a human and philanthropic enterprise would be permitted to function by the bureaucracies of either country today. In any case the ladies of the British Colony, including Lady Georgina's daughter Meriel worked diligently in the bandaging room — they didn't come out of sterilised packets in those days. As for Lady Georgina herself, 'she comes every morning, putting her hand to any work from bedmaking to washing clothes, to bringing the soldiers flowers or presents or taking parties out for motor rides'. She also gave to every outgoing soldier articles of clothing for himself, his wife and children.

One sentence in Miss St Clair's article makes strange reading today: 'It is quite pathetic to see 30 or 40 convalescents standing up in the dining hall, leaning on their crutches and facing the sacred ikon to sing their grace before meals and which is taken from the 145th Psalm: "The eyes of all wait upon Thee, O Lord, and Thou givest them their meat in due season. Thou openest Thine hand and fillest all things living with plenteousness". After supper they also say the Lord's Prayer, a hymn and the National Anthem.' Which curiously enough bore a striking resemblance to God Save The King:

---

[9] *The British Hospital Petrograd,* Janet St Clair. *The Nursing Times,* 18th September 1915. It was also known as the King George V Hospital.

God protect the Tsar!
Powerful and Sovereign
Reign to our glory,
To our glory;
Reign to the terror of our enemies,
Oh, Orthodox Tsar!
God protect the Tsar!

Hearing it sung by 100 *sanitars* at sunset in the Dvinsk forest, Lady Sybil wrote in her diary that it was the loveliest anthem in the world.

There is another sentence, tucked into the middle of this account of Lady Georgina's hospital, which caught my eye. 'The expected arrival in this country in October of a British Hospital Unit is interesting the British Colony here . . .' No doubt; for Sir George had been instructed to find accommodation for the Anglo-Russian Hospital and it was clear that this would put his wife's personal accomplishment in the shade. One may sympathise with her and perhaps it was fortunate that Lady Muriel didn't arrive in the first place because when she did so, six months later, they immediately quarrelled. So it is to Lady Sybil that the credit should be given for establishing the very best relations with this somewhat formidable woman. Perhaps Sir George helped in smoothing the path between the two competing enterprises. Not that Lady Georgina gave in easily. When organising a soirée for the medical and nursing staff, she drew the line at VAD's; and was considerably affronted to find that one of these, no doubt herself a lady of rank, had been invited to tea with the Tsarina on a day when she herself had been to tea with the Grand Duchess.

It may seem a strange coincidence that my three Ladies were all the daughters of Earls. Lady Georgina was doubtless involved because of her husband; but the other two achieved this of their own free wills, because of what they considered they ought to do in the circumstances. Having set their minds to the task they did not falter and being of course unpaid, they felt not only an obligation but an urge to see the whole thing through. They were brave, though probably no more so than many others; but I also believe they had a kind of inborn feeling of leadership which devolved from their families' backgrounds. It may not be agreeable to some to use such an argument today but I think that this may explain why these two remarkable women accomplished what they did.

25

Two photographs exist which include all my three Ladies. One, which is reproduced, shows the Tsarina and her four daughters when they attended the ceremony of the Blessing of the Field Hospital. The other appeared in the London *Sketch* on 28th June 1916 on the occasion of the presentation of two motor-ambulances to the hospital by Queen Alexandra. Seated on each side of the Grand Duchess Marie Pavlovna Vladimir in the front row of the group are Lady Sybil and Lady Muriel. Behind stands Lady Georgina almost extinguished in furs and with her, Dr Fleming, the Matron and WDH. At each extremity of the group are figures of immense dignity: to the right, Prince Toumanoff the Military Chief of Petrograd, bearing a magnificent forked beard; to the left, His Majesty's Ambassador resplendent in black top hat, monocle, wing-collar and gold-headed cane. Those were the days.

Outward Bound

In mid October the advance party set out from Newcastle upon Tyne in the Norwegian ship *Irma,* whose name was prominently displayed and illuminated on both sides of the upper deck. The possibility of German submarines worried them but at least they were on a neutral boat. The passage to Stavanger was without incident and later on so many people went this way to Russia that it became a well-guarded convoy route. The party consisted of Lady Sybil, 'Countess Olga [presumably the Grand Duchess Olga of Oldenburg], Mr Ian Malcolm MP and the newly appointed Commandant, Dr Fleming. Their instruction from the London Committee was to find accommodation in Petrograd for the hospital. Having crossed Norway, Sweden and Finland by train they had a 'red carpet' reception in Petrograd and were met by Major-General Sir John Hanbury-Williams, the Head of the British Military Mission and a personal friend of the Tsar, and by representatives of the British Embassy and of the Russian Red Cross — an indication of the importance which both countries attached to this initiative. In Stockholm even the austere Foreign Minister Mr Wallenstein had received them at luncheon, 'the second time only that I have lunched at home in two years', as he remarked.

Lady Sybil's diary records something of the journey along the northern shore of the Gulf of Finland where the railway line runs between the sea and the endless silver birch forests; and I do not think it can have been much different from the same journey which my wife and I took from Helsinki to Leningrad in 1965. Indeed we might very well have travelled in the same train with its anti-macassars and lace curtains. In one of his letters WDH remarked that 'the broad gauge and slow speed makes travel by train in Russia very comfortable and pleasant'. Certainly our own train never exceeded 40 mph and I imagine that the neat farmsteads in the forest clearings which we saw must have looked very much the same to them in 1915 except that now, on the Russian side of the border, the forest has been scorched and totally evacuated, so as to leave nothing except wire, watchtowers, tank-traps and gun-emplacements.

Lady Sybil's account ended with these words: 'We still don't know whether our hospital has been offered to the Red Cross or us? What shall we find?' It really does seem quite extraordinary that they knew so little about what they were going to try to do. Maybe that is why she added, 'Pray for me'.

The main party followed some three weeks later by the longer and incidentally less dangerous route around the North Cape to Archangel. They sailed in the SS *Calypso,* a ship of 2876 grt from London on 30th October and made Archangel successfully, probably about 6th November; the last ship, it is said, to do so before the winter ice closed the White Sea until the following Spring. In peacetime the *Calypso* had traded out of the east coast of England to Norway, the Baltic and North Russia. Designed to carry 12 passengers in addition to freight, she had been converted to accommodate nearly 1,000 personnel; 57 first class, 44 second class and 863 third class. My cousin Sir Frederic Harmer, sometime Deputy Chairman of the P&O Steam Navigation Co discovered this remarkable piece of information and in a letter to me he added: 'If you tried that on battery hens nowadays, the RSPCA would prosecute'. The *Calypso* was subsequently on Admiralty service as an armed merchant cruiser, a prison ship and at other times carrying refugees. Unhappily she was torpedoed off Flamborough Head in July 1916 with the loss of 30 lives.

Miss Mary MacDonald, a nurse who travelled in this same ship presented an album of snapshots many years later to the BRCS and among these there is a photograph, taken from the bridge, of the lane through the ice-floes by which they approached Archangel. Men stand on the firmer ice on either side of the lane carrying long poles, presumably to stop the floes from freezing up. Reaching Archangel they were warmly received by the Russian Guard (wrote Blunt) who dined them well, and informed them that owing to congestion upon the railways they would have to remain in Archangel for at least three weeks. They were appalled, particularly the nurses, who said that every hour of delay was costing Russian lives. The British jute agent, a certain Captain 'Sandy' Proctor and known locally as the King of Archangel came to their rescue and they got away in three days. WDH said in later years that it took a good deal of bribery to accomplish this feat.

That was not the end of their troubles. The route from Archangel to Petrograd was long and devious, as a look at the map will show. By contrast Murmansk, an ice-free port for the greater part of the year, lay almost due north of Petrograd, a distance of about 700 miles and was connected directly by railway to that city. This seaport had only been constructed in 1915 as an allied supply depôt for the Eastern Front and was scarcely operational at the time so they had to use the railway which went southwards from Archangel almost as far as Moscow, before their train could turn west for Petrograd, a total distance of some 1,240 miles. At the junction of Yaroslavl they again found themselves shunted into a siding and from this they once more had to extricate themselves in the appropriate manner. They reached Petrograd at 4 a.m. in the morning of either the 14th or 1st November, according to the Old Style (OS) calendar which Russia was still using and which was 13 days 'behind' Western Europe.

The four chief doctors left England on 24th November, ten days after the arrival of the main party, the assumption being that they would be able to move into a hospital prepared for them and ready to receive casualties. The surgeons, Waterhouse and WDH, the physician Gould May and the radiologist Flavelle travelled on an afternon train from Kings Cross to Newcastle upon Tyne to board the SS *Iris* for Bergen. During the journey there occured an incident which WDH recorded in detail in his diary:

> At about 5.45 asked by Guard to see a man who was supposed to have shot himself. Found him lying on seat of carriage — very pale — pulseless — slightly restless but conscious. About one pint of blood on floor. Found wound in posterior part of left axilla: haemorrhage apparently stopped. Gave him a drink of water and took down his name and address. Patient very faint, said he was sitting reading his newspaper and didn't know what had happened.

What had happened was that a drunken soldier in the next compartment had fired his rifle and then thrown it out of the window. The bullet passed through the partition, then through the patient's armpit, no doubt injuring the main axillary blood vessels and was later found in the next compartment to that. Now few things are more difficult to stop than an express train when it is proceeding, so to speak, *ventre à terre*. After a consultation, a message wrapped around a

29

potato was thrown out at an intermediate station and the express was signalled down at Selby. The casualty was disembarked after the other doctors had agreed that nothing further could be done until he reached hospital. The diary continues:

> Offered to go with him but Station-master refused to delay train; impossible to leave it therefore as under orders for Petrograd. Handed slip of paper with man's name address and statements to Guard of train.

His name and address are also recorded in the diary and the very first letter which WDH received from home told him that the soldier had died the same night. It is not known what happened to the soldier who shot him.

Also on the train was a Miss Bates. It was my belief that she might possibly have been the Matron of the hospital and my reasons for thinking so are given in a later chapter. In the event I was proved wrong. The party had a miserable crossing to Bergen and continued in what can only be described as a rather leisurely manner to Christiania (Oslo) where they stayed at the Grand Hotel — 'full of Germans!'; and then on to Stockholm — 'tea with Crown Princess'; and around the Gulf of Bothnia to Haporanda, which lies on the west bank of the river separating Sweden from Finland and Russia. They walked across the ice in 36 degrees of frost to Tornio and, although their train had reached Haporanda at nine in the morning and their *laissez-passer* had got them through the Swedish Customs without difficulty, it was after 8 p.m. before they cleared the Russian Customs and were able to entrain for Petrograd. It was figuratively and literally a chilly welcome. The severity of the winter of 1915-16 has been briefly mentioned but according to WDH's diary 'the Russian Govt. didn't warn other countries of early winter — coldest for 100 years. Probably 100 ships drifting in White Sea, many of them without food. Doubtful whether they can ever be found by icebreakers'.

One of these ships was of great concern to the hospital. The stores and equipment were following hard on the heels of the *Calypso* (if such an analogy may be permitted in a maritime context) in a ship called the *Abaris*. Also on passage from the Tyne at about the same time was the *Arabis*. One got stuck in the ice; the other was damaged in heavy seas and had to return to England for repairs. No one was quite sure which was which and this doubt prevailed for a surprisingly long time. Thus WDH, on 29th November OS: 'The hospital is nearing completion but I fear that we shall not get to work yet as the stores are icebound and no one knows when they will be recovered'. On 6th December he wrote: 'The mystery about the stores gets worse every day. Yours of 2nd December [English date] says they are still in England. A week ago we wired to know if we were to buy a new lot here and today a reply has come saying do nothing for a fortnight'. In fact the *Arabis* had succeeded in reaching Archangel and it was the *Abaris,* together with the stores, which disappeared into the ice. In the event then they had to start from scratch in re-equipping their hospital. The precious and valuable stores did not reach them for a further five months though by that time the staff was busily engaged and found them of immense value.

The Doctors

The Commandant, Dr Andrew Fleming CMG had been selected from a considerable number of applicants by the Committee because he had proved himself a capable and successful hospital administrator in Southern Rhodesia. A Scot and 45 years of age, he was well qualified for the post, having the FRCS (England) and the DPM (Cambridge). He was something of an autocrat and though he prided himself on always asking the opinions of his staff, his critics maintained that he had invariably made up his mind in advance of what was best and was determined to assert his authority. Since he was dealing with a group of volunteers rather than servicemen, this approach did not work out too well and there was inevitably considerable discord. Both Lady Muriel and Lady Sybil liked him, though both admitted that they found him difficult to work with. Shortly after her arrival in Russia Lady Sybil wrote home: 'I like Dr Fleming immensely. He has a great sense of humour. We are very goods friends'. But within a few weeks she had the distressing task of requesting his resignation, requiring the help of Mr Waterhouse in so doing. The fact was that about this time the senior staff told Lady Sybil that 'unless something is done about Fleming we will all go home'; and this, it must be supposed, they had the right to do.

Whether the senior staff had a Contract with the A-R H. Committee is uncertain but the doctors who went out later on certainly did. Among Sir Geoffrey Jefferson's papers was his own Agreement, a thoroughly legal document, declaring *Whereby It Is Agreed As Follows* . . . etc. In brief this two-page document laid down the terms of employment 'for a certain period (subject as hereinafter mentioned) of six calendar months as from the date of departure from England and thereafter the said employment shall (at the option of the Committee) be continued from month to month for the duration of the war subject to determination by one calendar month's previous notice to be given by either party to the other'. There followed clauses about what should happen if the war ended prematurely — an unlikely event to be sure — and stating that the salary was £400 per annum; and that uniform, passage to and from Russia and accommodation would be provided by the Committee. The final clause of the Agreement is of interest. 'Should the Surgeon object to perform any duties for which the Representative of the Committee for the time being in Russia may think the Surgeon qualified or should the Representative . . . for any reason whatever consider the Surgeon unsuitable owing to ill-health or any other cause then it shall be competent for the said Representative . . . to forthwith terminate this Agreement and thereupon this Agreement shall become absolutely void and the Surgeon shall not be entitled to any claim against the Committee or any members thereof in respect of salary, board and lodging or otherwise.'

Tough stuff, it may be thought! But wise in the event, for it enabled both Lady Sybil and Lady Muriel to replace (I will not say dismiss) several doctors whom they felt were not able to carry out their duties to the hospital in the months to come.

As for Dr Fleming, Contract or no, he reacted well. To his credit he offered to give up the post of Commandant and 'go into the wards under Waterhouse and Gould May'. A way out of the difficulty was found when Lady Muriel arrived in April the following year and he went off with her to arrange the organisation of Field Hospitals behind the front around Kiev. During July we will find him assisting WDH in operations at Lutsk and Rovno.

Unhappily the friction remained and eventually, for the general benefit of all, he returned to England. He showed no resentment and indeed generously wrote the words with which I end my chapter on Materia Medica.

WDH must have agreed I think, because on 29th August he wrote to my mother: 'Fleming is starting [for England] to-morrow and I shall feel rather lost as I have seen a great deal of him and there is no one else left. If you are in town go and see him and have him to a meal. He is a very nice fellow and has had a devil of a time here. Most of the staff have done their damnest to make things difficult and their disloyalty has done no good to the hospital. In spite of it all he has organised two excellent hospitals and they have done some good work'.

Mr H. F. Waterhouse MD, FRCS was 51.[1] The *Lives of the Fellows* of the Royal College of Surgeons describes him as 'a rapid and dextrous surgeon, impatient of delay, quick to distinguish the useful from the valueless, somewhat too enthusiastic and with little capacity for sustained interest or tedious back-work'. With what may seem somewhat brutal honesty this Dictionary of Surgical Biography continues: 'As a man Waterhouse was a good type of the English surgeon of his generation; tall, good-looking, courteous in manner, easy to address and a fluent speaker; being possessed of ample means he wrote but little'. To him however must be given the credit for introducing iodine-in-spirit as a skin preparation before operations, a method which largely replaced the more elaborate ones then in current use. At this time he was the Senior Surgeon to Charing Cross Hospital where he excelled as a teacher of both systematic and clinical surgery. He was a member of the Council of the Royal College of Surgeons and an examiner for at least five Universities. Volunteering for the Anglo-Russian Hospital he was appointed Surgeon-in-Chief (with WDH as his 'number two') and spent 11 months in Russia. He spoke French fluently and acquired more Russian than any of his colleagues. It was written of him that 'to the wounded he was always sympathetic and they accepted his advice without hesitation'. Maybe he was a trifle conceited, for it is on record that he described himself to a Russian colleague as one of the best seven surgeons in London. (Unhappily history is silent as to the identity of the other six.) He and WDH worked very amicably together though he didn't get on too well with Lady Muriel when she arrived to take charge in the Spring of '16; and it is clear that he got on very badly indeed with Fleming. This became evident during the hiatus when Lady Sybil was organising the Dmitri hospital and when there was no medical work to be done. Lady Muriel, still at home, was in one of her grandiose moods and she telegraphed the hapless Dr Fleming: 'Committee Waterhouse Harmer think important follow original scheme have hospital 400 beds fed eventually by three field hospitals understand suggested base incapable further expansion urge acquiring additional building'. Whether Waterhouse and WDH had discussed this idea with their Commandant is not known but it hardly had the effect of improving

---

[1] Later Sir Herbert Waterhouse Kt 1917. He died in 1931 aged 67, following an unfortunate accident the previous year when two motor cars collided alongside the pavement on which he was walking, injuring him gravely. He was awarded his Knighthood for his services to the A-R H.

relations on the spot. Lady Muriel got into the same sort of trouble the following summer when she was at Lutsk. During bitter fighting and facing terrible casualties, she cabled Lord Cheylesmore demanding the immediate despatch of 100 ambulances. Neither these nor the transport for them were available of course, let alone the money to acquire them.

On this occasion however Lady Sybil was in no doubt. Advised by Sir George Buchanan she replied that any request for a second building, before the first had even been opened or any proof given of its value, would be highly injudicious.

Douglas Harmer MC (Cantab), FRCS was the Senior Surgeon to the hospital. His degree rates more than a footnote. I have a letter from him written in 1960 in which he stated that he was the thirteenth holder of this degree and the first to achieve it by examination, his predecessors having had it granted *honoris causa*. The truth is that in 1901 he applied to take the degree by examination and this seems to have caused something of a flurry in the Medical Faculty at Cambridge because there were no examiners who were willing — or even able, since they were mostly physicians — to set the papers. The matter was satisfactorily resolved: he sat and passed, and in the succeeding years another half dozen or so surgeons acquired it, including his own brother-in-law J. P. Hedley, who must surely rank amongst the most highly qualified doctors of his time.[2]

The introduction of the Military Cross in December 1914 placed the University in some difficulty. Although officers who were awarded the decoration were not officially entitled to put the initials MC after their names, it soon became customary to do so. Consequently the many RAMC doctors who received the Military Cross appeared to be Masters of Surgery. In 1916 the Council of the Senate bowed to the inevitable and decreed in the University Ordinances that the degrees of BC and MC should become BCh and MCh (subsequently BChir and MChir). This did not please those who already held the MC and at one point it was seriously suggested that they should sue the University for 'wrongful designation'. However, the most militant of the Masters died and the others, who were doing more useful things in the war, accepted that it would not be right to press the point. 'We had a

---

[2] Had it been in existence he might also have qualified for *The Guinness Book of Records.* John Prescot Hedley MA, MB, MC, MD, FRCP, FRCS, FRCOG, Consultant Obstetrician and Gynaecologist to St Thomas's Hospital.

meeting (my father wrote) and decided to have a bit of fun: we agreed on condition that we could wear red gowns like the Doctors of Medicine. We didn't get far with our demand and actually agreed that it was quite reasonable'. Nevertheless and quite properly, he continued to write MC (Cantab) on his surgical papers; and when the editors of journals corrected this in proof to MChir he answered in scathing terms! In 1960 the Clerk to the Registrary replied to my enquiry that my father was indeed the sole survivor of the old degree. Thus he was both first and last: in a sense alpha and omega.

How WDH joined the staff has already been told. As everyone knows, time and tide wait for no man and in fact he quite literally almost missed the boat. After the excitement of the shot soldier, he had dined with his father-in-law Dr John Hedley, who was a General Practitioner in Middlesbrough, at the Station Hotel in Newcastle. It must have been a good dinner, because although the *Iris* did not sail until midnight, he had the greatest difficulty in finding a taxi to take him to the docks and the gangway was in the process of being raised as he arrived to board her.

Two young doctors also sailed with the main complement. One was a Captain Mark Gardner MD, RAMC who came from the Australian Hospital in Boulogne: of him I know nothing except that he returned to England the following July because he considered there wasn't anything for him to do. 'And I can't say I blame him', wrote WDH. 'There is no doubt he is wasting his time here, *as we all are* [My italics. Within a few weeks they were up to their necks in it] but it is very annoying not to have given us more notice and I am left alone now with no one but a dentist and a dresser to help me.' This surprising ability for the staff, both senior and junior, to be able to pack up and go home when they felt so inclined continues to be a matter for remark, for although actually the official tour-of-duty was six months it seems to have been very liberally interpreted.

The other was Mr H. Q. F. Thompson, a young doctor who came from St George's Hospital though he does not seem to have qualified there. Of him also I wish I was able to say more. WDH regarded him highly — 'he is a very nice lad' — and he is noteworthy for two reasons: first, he remained with the hospital longer than any of the other surgeons who went out with the original team and second, and by far the more important, it is recorded that during the four-day battle around Kirli-Baba in the Carpathians, he treated over 400

36

casualties with no other assistance and under appalling conditions. For this he received the Cross of St George the following Christmas. In the matter of decorations, the Russians awarded the Cross of St George (not to be confused with our George Cross) and the Medal of St George. Lady Muriel was herself given the latter medal, second class, after the Battle of the River Stokhod. Legend has it that the most famous recipient was a cow who charged a German aeroplane which had made a forced landing at Lutsk.

Of the doctors who joined the staff of the Anglo-Russian Hospital later, none was destined to become as distinguished as Mr Geoffrey Jefferson.[3] His first post after qualification had been that of house-surgeon to Mr Waterhouse at Tite Street Children's Hospital. His future wife, who was Canadian and who was also a doctor, had done her pre-clinical work at the Royal Free Hospital having qualified in Manchester: and it was there that they had met. In the first year of the war Jefferson was in British Columbia visiting his in-laws but feeling dissatisfied with his lot. In consequence he wrote to Waterhouse who suggested that he came to Russia: and there he went, arriving at the end of April 1916 and returning to England some 16 months later. At the age of 29 he had the MS (London) and FRCS (England) and an interest in what was a comparatively new speciality, neurosurgery. He spent the summer and autumn of 1916 at Rovno, Lutsk and Kiev, places which will feature prominently in succeeding chapters and the remainder of his time at the Base Hospital in Petrogràd. His achievements will be recorded later and amongst these was the removal of a bullet from the cerebellum of an 18 year-old Tartar soldier, a remarkable accomplishment for those days. On the eve of his departure from Russia, he wrote: 'Until the war is over I'm sure I couldn't rest unless doing war work and I do want to join the RAMC or the CMAC.' He did. He was put in charge of the Cranial Surgery Unit at the British Hospital at Wimereux in Belgium and it was here, one must suppose, that he began the career which was to lead to him becoming one of the outstanding neurosurgeons of the world.

While working at Lutsk he was given a Fabergé cigarette-case by an admiring aristocratic Russian liaison officer, inscribed: *'En souvenir de Lutsk et de tout ce que s'est passé de gai, de triste et de macabre'.* Among Sir

---

[3] Later Sir Geoffrey Jefferson Kt 1950, Fellow of the Royal Society and the recipient of at least a dozen Honorary Degrees from Universities in Britain and overseas. Professor of Neurosurgery in the University of Manchester, he died in 1961 aged 75.

Geoffrey's *Selected Papers* in the library of the Royal College of Surgeons there is one written in 1956 and entitled *Return to Russia*. In this he recalls the incident: 'What was so gay? There was more than enough sadness of course. Of the macabre, perhaps an episode related to Douglas Harmer and myself one night in Kiev by Baron A. (let us call him), a member of a famous family and a Colonel of a Guard's cavalry regiment, may suffice:'

In recent fighting his regiment had had its first really satisfactory set-to with German cavalry and had routed them. He had celebrated by handing out three bottles of brandy. Afterwards our Baron had gone out with some of this precious stuff to see if any of his wounded men had been overlooked. As he walked his horse beside a copse his eye was caught by the weak movements of a figure lying at the edge of the trees, yet there was a glint of metal. He went on; 'I have eyes like a cat, I can see in the dark, I could see that the man was a wounded German officer who was going to shoot me. I threw myself from my horse and pounced on him taking him by the throat. I said, *"Guten Abend, mein Lieber* — you are a brave man, you are wounded and yet you wish to kill me. I respect you. But, for myself, I have no wish to die. I have a wife whom I love, a wife who loves me, so I prefer to live. Since I cannot trust you, it is you who must die." So I grasped his neck and I said, *"Gute Nacht"* — and crack! he was dead!' It was an impressive tale by so powerfully built yet so cultured a man, so incongruous an anecdote as we sat peacefully that evening eating wild strawberries in the open interior courtyard of a Kiev hotel, after walking in the gardens of the Merchants' Club on a cliff at the city's edge.

Jefferson was also given the Medal of St George for his work at Lutsk and it is sad to record that both this and the Fabergé cigarette-case were stolen from his wife's luggage in Sweden on her way home from Russia. A man of such keen intellect naturally formed his own opinions about the other doctors on the staff and some of these are noted in Chapter 9. Officially he remained discreet. It seems that Lady Muriel may have asked him what he thought of some of his seniors because we find him writing to her from Lutsk: '. . . but really it's so difficult to do so: much of the amusement arises out of the personalities of some of my colleagues and it isn't easy to transfer this to paper'. In the same letter he apologised for being unable to send her an apparently promised account of the activities of his unit after the Battle of the Stokhod: but he did so later with Fleming, in a report to the London Committee and this will be mentioned again in due course.

Two other surgeons involved in the work of the hospital should be mentioned. Mr Charles Jennings Marshall MS, FRCS was surgical registrar to Mr Waterhouse and at 26 years of age he went out with Jefferson, five nurses, two VADs, Miss Jameson and Lady Muriel herself. Later he replaced his chief when he returned to England in the autumn of '16. On his arrival WDH had some doubts about him but he proved himself in the event and combined with both of them in what seems to have been the only general medical paper published concerning the work of the A-R H. Of his activities in Russia I have been able to discover virtually nothing but he remained there for something like six or nine months and on his return joined the RAMC and went off to Salonika. After the war he was appointed Orthopaedist to King's College Hospital but resigned this post in order to take up general surgery at 'The Cross'.

Mr Stephen Paget — no relation of Sir Richard's — took the place of WDH when he left for home in October 1916. The appointment seems to have surprised my father. 'I would never have thought of Paget' he noted, though the rumour that Sir Arthur William Mayo Robson, Vice-President of the Royal College of Surgeons and 63 years of age, might be coming out alarmed him to the extent of adding two exclamation marks in his diary. Paget was the youngest son of the famous Sir James Paget Bt whose eponym is still attached to the condition called osteitis deformans.[4] Though he was less than 60 at the time, Lady Sybil — this slip of a girl! — appears to have considered him antediluvian. 'We have given old Mr Paget notice', she wrote to Lady Muriel in January 1917. 'Poor old man, I did feel sorry for him — especially as he and Flavelle loathed each other and Flavelle was not the most tactful in the things he said. He was really rather too old and his health not sufficiently good for the job. Of course Flavelle was an ass to bring him out. I must say he has been charming to me about it. I enclose his letter.' What Paget actually wrote in that letter was this: 'Everybody has been amazingly kind and friendly to me. I love being here but it won't be too bad to get home when the time comes'. Sad as

---

[4] Paget's disease of Bone. There is also Paget's disease of the Nipple (a pre-cancerous breast lesion) and Paget's Recurrent fibroid. James Paget 1814-1899. Surgeon to St Bartholomew's Hospital, where a ward is named after him.

any surgical biographer must feel to read such an assessment of a colleague, it is impossible not to admire the authority of his Commanding Officer. Thus Mr Stephen Paget MS, FRCS, surgeon to the Middlesex Hospital, leaves my story.

There was also an anaesthetist, Dr G. A. Jones, who was on the staff of St Mark's Hospital and the Samaritan Hospital for Women. There is a photograph of this young man standing at the head of a portable operating table while Waterhouse and WDH are at work on a patient's injured arm. Dr Fleming looks on while two nurses, red crosses prominent on their aprons, deal with the instruments. It is somewhat shaming to have to admit that in those days anaesthetists were regarded as somewhat second-class medical citizens and so, although WDH described him as 'quite the best of the bunch', Dr Jones receives no other mention by name in any of the papers I have consulted except that which lists him amongst the original staff. In those days anaesthetists 'gave stuff' (and were therefore colloquially known as Stuffists) and their Art was confied to the chloroform mask and the 'rag and bottle' method of administering ether. 'Gas' was sufficient for operations of brief duration but was quite impractical for use in the field hospitals, where indeed many of the wounded had to be operated upon without any anaesthetic at all. It is very different to-day when a team of anaesthetists, presiding over banks of electronically controlled medico-physiological apparatus, are almost the most important persons at a major operation.[5]

That I have said nothing so far about the physicians attached to the hospital should not be construed as a mark of disrespect; for as everyone knows, physicians are of an altogether Higher Order of Beings than surgeons. Yet it is a fact that a war hospital is basically a surgical hospital.

The first prospectus published by the London Committee stated that the Physician to the Hospital was Dr T. J. Horder.[6] In fact he never went to Russia and was actually advised not to do so by WDH on at least two occasions on the grounds that his talents would be

---

[5] 'So-and-so stuffs for me', my father would say. But at the Royal Society of Medicine (it is said) an anaesthetist was recently overheard saying to a colleague: 'I have eight surgeons working for me now'.

[6] Thomas Jeeves Horder MD, FRCP, GCVO 1918; Bt 1923; Baron Horder of Ashford 1933. 1871-1955.

wasted. None the less he continued to advise the Committee in London and sometimes in a manner which seems to have upset those on the job. 'I see a note in the *Lancet* (wrote WDH in April 1916) saying he cannot leave England and is representing us there. Miss Pearce [the secretary of the Committee] thinks differently but she is not the first person to complain about his ways. He is a troublesome person and I don't know why everyone runs after him so much.' No one who remembers 'Tommy' Horder will need reminding of his energy and enthusiasm for causes with which he wished to be associated. At a dinner in Lord Horder's honour (at which I was present) that superb orator, Mr Arthur Dickson Wright said of him: 'He will look after you from the cradle to the grave. As Chairman of the Family Planning Association he will see you into the world — unless his membership of the Abortion Society prevents your entry. He will guide your childhood through the NSPCC, nourish your adult education through his association with the Arts and Music, cherish you in old age through the Distressed Gentlefolk's Association and the Anti-noise League and see you to a comfortable end in his capacity as President of the London Cremation Society. But even then he will continue to look after your interests as Chairman of the Smoke Abatement Society'.

In his place there went Dr Gould May MD, MRCP[7] from the Middlesex Hospital. Most of his time was spent in Petrograd where there was much to do amongst the wounded and convalescents, because pneumonia and other infections were all too common and of course antibacterial and antibiotic drugs were then unknown. He and his like had the task of nursing them back to life after the surgeons had done their best. Few of the other physicians have left much imprint in the records. The 'useless' Doctor Williams has already been summarily dismissed in Chapter 3 by Lady Sybil and there was also 'Old Doctor Sevier who is useful and who we would keep — he knows Russian and is sensible'.

There was however one other as well, a Dr (or Professor) Graham Aspland who had been a medical missionary in China before the war. Oddly enough his wife had been my mother's governess and became a family friend. She qualified as a trained nurse, had worked with

[7] Subsequently Sir Gould May. He was associated with both Sir Thomas Horder and WDH in the treatment of the Prime Minister Mr Bonar Law in 1923, and it was for this service that he received his Knighthood. 'A most charming fellow (according to Jefferson), thin red face, most deeply lined.'

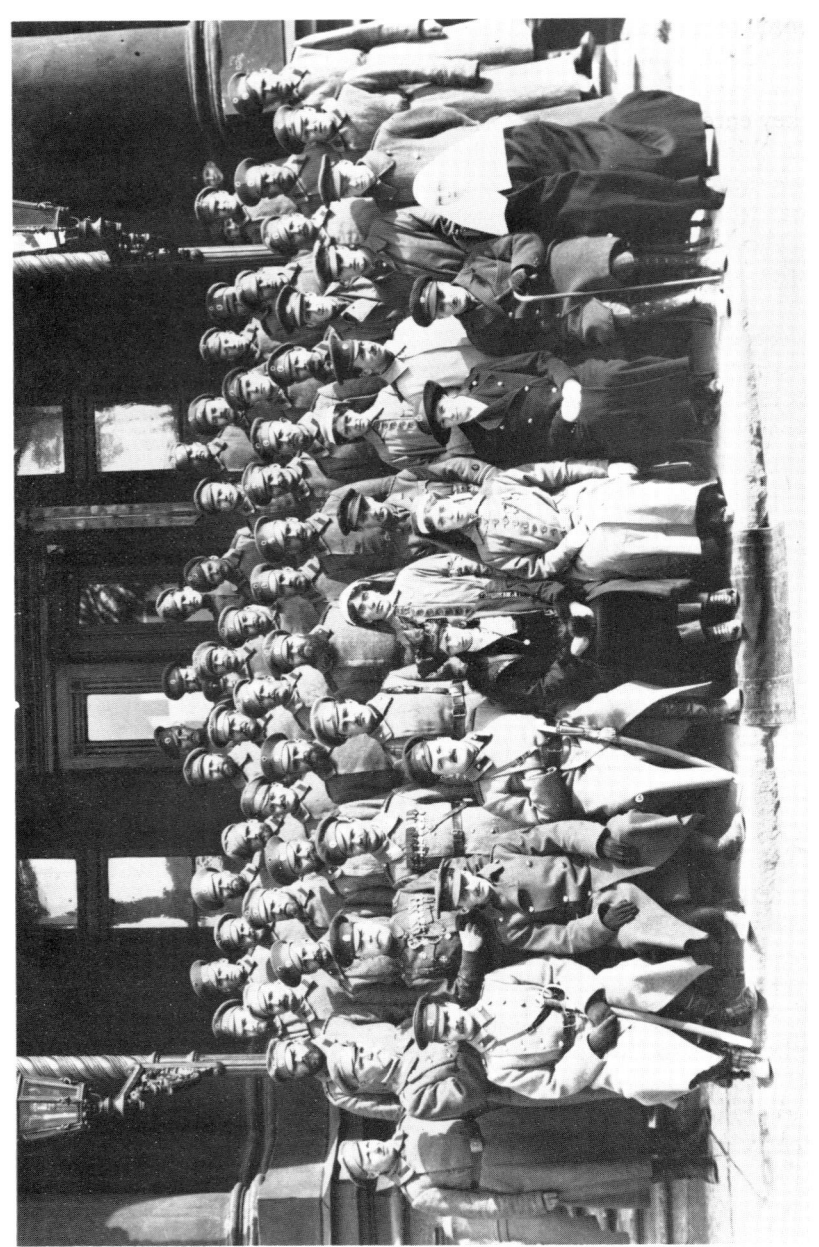

THE HOSPITAL STAFF

Grenfell in Labrador and nursed in Peking. But she did not accompany her husband to Russia. He had transferred his activities, apparently on his own initiative, to Tiflis in the Caucasus at about the time when Turkey entered the war on Germany's side and a new front was opened up in this area, believing that he might be of help to the Armenians. There seems to have been little to do however and in July 1916 there is a note from WDH: 'I have just received a letter from Aspland who says they have failed to find any pressing work and suggesting he should join us'. So up he came to Volhynia, a mere 1300 miles or so, at the drop of a telegram from WDH. What a wonderful war! And very good he was too: so much so that, when Fleming left for home and a new Commandant was needed, it was Aspland who was favoured by most of the staff.

However, the job went to Dr John Flavelle, Radiologist at St Bartholomew's Hospital, and who (as already noted) was one of the four specialists who went to Petrograd to set up the hospital. A man of private means, he had given an ambulance to the French and had driven it himself in the Vosges during the first year of the war. He was also a Vice-President of the All English Tennis Club and had served in the Boer War. So it is understandable perhaps that he found it difficult to take orders from others. However that may be, it is necessary to remind the reader that diagnostic radiology was at that time almost in its infancy. One of the things upon which the Anglo-Russian Hospital Committee prided itself was being able to send two X-ray machines to Petrograd: and the fact that they were stuck in the ice in the *Abaris* for nearly six months was a bitter blow at the time. They were designed to be mobile and although of immense weight by to-day's standards it was found possible to deploy them in the field hospitals, where they were of tremendous help in locating foreign bodies in the tissues of injured men. Dr Flavelle must have been gratified that he obtained replacements just in time for the Official Blessing of the Hospital and was able to see them liberally sprinkled with Holy Water by the Bishop. Like most of the staff who it is my duty to describe, John Flavelle seems to have been an opinionated man. Having had the good fortune to marry a rich wife he was able to take up the new speciality of radiology, which in those days was less rewarding than it subsequently became, and also to indulge his belief in the Theory of Socialism — he seems to have been an admirer of Lenin by all accounts. WDH found him 'the most argumentative devil I have ever lived with and as he always works himself up into a frenzy it is difficult to know how to take him. Otherwise he has many good points. He is very keen on the music here and goes to something, concert or opera, once or twice each week'.

That he was made Commandant is perhaps surprising considering that he was described as being 'the biggest autocrat professing democratic principles that I ever met' (by Lady Muriel): and that 'his arrogance is only surpassed by his impudence or vice versa' (by Lady Sybil). Moreover he had returned to England at the end of his six months tour-of-duty but was recalled to take up the appointment. They would have preferred WDH himself.

Lady Sybil (Petrograd) to Lady Muriel (London).

January 31 1917.

Flavelle wishes to be home by the 21st of April English Date. I am glad and would not encourage him to stay. I think he is good in some things like the motor column. I think he got them all into line and they were all frightened of him — excellent for them — but he is not liked by any of the Russians. His inability to understand or speak a single word of either French or Russian puts him at a great disadvantage and he is far too excitable and *entêté* when he gets an idea into his head.

In one of your letters you spoke of Harmer possibly coming out [again]. In many ways I think he would do admirably. He speaks French (a really necessary thing for a C.O. I think) and he now understands a very great deal of Russian. The Russians all like him and he is always dignified. I heard a Russian was talking of our different C.O.'s the other day and said — he liked Fleming and Harmer very much — but that the present man [Flavelle] looked exactly like a Russian peasant. I thought that would rather amuse you because he does look rather like that sometimes when he hasn't shaved in the morning and his hair and eyes are more than usually wild.

Harmer's fault is perhaps that he is rather weak but I think his other qualities outweigh this. He is a good surgeon and knows how things should be done. I must say I should be delighted to hear that Harmer was coming and unless you have an exceptionally good man in view I think it would be well worth the Committee making it worth Harmer's while to come.

It appears that they tried to do so, though WDH did not fall for the bait. He had in fact acted for a short time as C.O. when Fleming was

44

on leave and the Committee now sent him a cheque for £200 on account of this. This was a considerable sum: the prospectus for the Appeal had stated that £100 would equip and maintain one bed in the hospital for one year. He replied:

Dear Lady Muriel Paget

I am very much obliged to you for your kind letter enclosing a cheque for £200 . . . As the whole period was only about a month I do not feel justified in accepting anything approaching £200 because it would obviously be unfair to my colleagues, some of whom have given just as much to the cause as I did. I shall be obliged if you will tell the Committee how much I appreciate their generosity . . .

Yours sincerely,

Ch. for £200 enclosed.   Douglas Harmer.

Before closing this account of the medical staff I must mention six flimsy, yellowing foolscap sheets of paper which were found by Pamela Lady Glenconner. They bear no heading but are clearly authentic and of historic interest since they list the entire Medical Staff, Nurses and VAD's, Orderlies, Chauffeurs and Secretaries [see Appendix 3]. Amongst the doctors there are some names which do not occur elsewhere; for instance Major Kent Hughes, Major J. G. Hunt and Captain W. B. Macdermott. I think these were probably seconded from the RAMC and three such officers appear, in that uniform, in one of the photographic groups of the hospital staff. Dr William Lingard, Dr Edward Rivera and Dr Aron Pastel defeat me. Mr Graham Bott and Mr Harrison were the dispensers or pharmacists.

It remains to name two other doctors. Dr Arthur Rosher, 'a young big chap of 32 from Charing Cross', was the Bacteriologist *(sic)* and if nothing else, he became an expert on gas-gangrene. He was one of the original medical team and among the last to leave. In fact I believe he served longer than any other doctor. Finally Dr Walter Yeld, the last Commandant, of whom more will be told in connexion with the exodus in 1918.

I fear that I may have given the impression in this chapter of a group of cantankerous doctors squabbling amongst themselves and only being controlled by two somewhat domineering women. I do not believe this was really so. Men and women tend to put their opinions, their troubles, their criticisms in writing while leaving unsaid or unrecorded the better aspects of the days. I think it should be remembered also that at that time people were more forthright in their remarks than they are today and that in any case many of my quotations are privileged and were never intended for publication when they were written.

So let us now pass to the gentler sex.

Ministering Angels

The previous chapter described the doctors who staffed the hospitals but *primus inter pares* in any hospital is the Matron. In this instance everyone who wrote about her agreed that she was superb. Hugh Walpole, who had been somewhat acid about Lady Georgina, became almost lyrical: 'I hear her praised on every side . . . this incomparable Matron . . .' Blunt confirms this also when writing of the disillusion of the nurses who, having arrived to tend the sick and wounded, found themselves at the Berlitz School of Languages trying to learn Russian and French while the hospital was being prepared for occupation. [French was then the second language in Russian. In fact it was the first language at the Imperial Court: and not so long before, German was spoken at Court in England and English at Court in Germany. Something no doubt to do with Queen Victoria.] Thus: 'Only the supreme tact of a supremely tactful Matron put a brake on something almost indistinguishable from a mutiny'. Tact seems to have been at a premium about this time because Walpole used the same word again soon after the official opening of the Hospital. 'I have been all over it and it is simply magnificent. I have seen so many hospitals and this beats them all. I hear it spoken of on every side. Lady Sybil's tact has been *immense* . . .'

There is no reason to doubt that these tributes were well deserved but without meaning to be churlish it has to be said that WDH in his letters and diary never comments upon the Matron's competence and indeed only mentions her on two occasions, first when she entrained to help set up the first field hospital and when she was present in the bunker in which Lady Sybil sustained her injury. To me the reason is clear: the staff of the best hospitals expected their matrons to be superb. But there was one quite extraordinary fact: I found it difficult to say with certainty who the Matron was. The Red Cross believed that it had been Miss Violetta Thurstan, and of her I will write more in due course. Blunt wrote that it was Miss Irvine Robertson but he mentions her by name once only and then in a footnote, referring to her elsewhere in his book simply as 'the Matron'. WDH never gave her a name at all and this was no doubt due to the peculiar British custom of identifying members of the nursing staff by their wards or departments, the former usually bearing the name of some famous doctor or benefactor of the hospital.

Even to-day a medical patient may find himself under the care of Sister Harvey, a surgical case under Sister Lister or (suitably enough) Sister Paget; and a name which may possibly still strike terror into the heart of any probationer nurse is Sister Tutor. In my own hospital this tradition was carried to extremes. Sister Throats and Sister Skins led their anonymous lives and the nurse who supervised the cleaners in the Outpatient department rejoiced in the astonishing name of Sister Scrubbers! To-day of course they are all Senior Deputy Assistant Nursing Officers . . . Matrons usually fared better for, although invariably addressed by title, most people at least knew their proper names. In this instance it does not seem to have been so. This at any rate is my excuse for being able to write so little about the 50 or more nurses who served the Anglo-Russian Hospitals.

There are two photographic groups of the hospital staff in which the Matron and the Assistant Matron are clearly seen, the former in respect of the position which she occupies in the front row. Both wear the same uniform and the Matron has a medal which appears to be that of the Cross of St George. Moreover she bears a striking resemblance to the picture in Miss McLaren's book[1] of Miss Violetta Thurstan; and this may be one of the reasons why the archivist of the BRCS believed that she was the Matron. Let me then examine Miss Thurstan's credentials.

Like all the women about whom I write, she too was exceptional. A London Hospital trained nurse, who was of somewhat frail health, she had been given charge of a convalescent home in Hythe in 1914. However soon after the outbreak of the war she persuaded the St John Ambulance Association to let her go to Brussels with a contingent of their nurses. Here she witnessed the historic entry of the German army into that city. An account reads: 'Some days later when the German authorities asked for volunteers to nurse at a little town called Marcelline near Charleroi, Miss Thurstan offered to go and took two nurses with her. Here she was in charge under German Military Command of Belgian, French and German wounded for some weeks

---

[1] *Women of the War.* Barbara McLaren. Hodder & Stoughton 1917.

under very trying conditions aggravated by the brutality of the German system of discipline even as regards their own wounded'. Later she collected her original nurses and took them by train through Germany to the Danish frontier, 'during which journey they were subjected to constant insult and humiliation, made up for by a cordial reception at Copenhagen'.

Hearing of the need for trained nurses in Russia she made her way to Petrograd and offered her services to the Russian Red Cross. Once again she witnessed the fall of a capital city, Warsaw; and helped in the evacuation of 18,000 wounded from Lodz in the short space of four days. Eventually she was wounded and returned to England bearing the Cross of St George 'for courage and devotion'. We read that 'having recovered from her wounds, in 1915 Miss Thurstan assisted in organising the hospital units which were being sent from England to work among the *refugees*' [my italics: not the wounded, be it noted]. There are references to mobile units but no mention at all of the Anglo-Russian Hospital as such. Reluctantly, I struck her off the list of possibilities but in doing so I record her own feelings. 'Verily the English language lacks words to express the suffering that these people underwent, and nothing that we can imagine would be worse than the reality.'

Then there was Miss Bates, the nurse who took the 2.30 p.m. train from King's Cross with the four senior medical staff and who no doubt comforted the unfortunate soldier who was mortally wounded on that occasion. It seemed possible that she might have been travelling to take up the appointment of Matron but a scrap of paper in the BRCS records eliminated this possibility. It was her Red Cross card on which is written: 'Nov. 2nd 1915, arrived Russia. May 4th 1916, will report home. Has been H. Sister — v. good and energetic'. From this it is clear that she went out to take charge of the Nurses Home which had been established on the Vladimirsky Prospekt about ten minutes walk from the Dmitri Palace. She was in fact the Assistant Matron. Another source speaks highly of the Home Sister and the manner in which she looked after her nurses. She may well have regretted that she was not there in March 1917 when her nurses had to run the gauntlet of the revolutionary mob in order to reach the Palace and their patients.

Eventually the identity of the Matron was proved in the simplest manner and as something of an anti-climax. Among Lady Muriel's papers there were three brochures prepared by the Committee of the

Anglo-Russian Hospital and two of these print her name. She was Miss S. S. Irvine Robertson. But even then it took me the best part of a year to discover much about her. Neither the Royal College of Nursing nor the General Nursing Council could trace her and this was in part due to the fact that a National Register of Nurses was not established until 1919. St Thomas's, St Bartholomew's, The London, The Middlesex and Charing Cross Hospitals all denied knowledge of her having trained with them. A chance reference in a letter suggested that it might have been the Royal Free Hospital but they too could not confirm this. Then quite unexpectedly a picture postcard of her arrived, sent me by her nephew,[2] and there on the bib of her uniform (though only visible through a magnifying glass) was the familiar shield — *party per pale argent and sable a chevron counter-changed* — the badge of the Royal Hospital of Saint Bartholomew.

Sophia Irvine Robertson was the daughter of the Reverend Alexander Irvine Robertson DD and came of a medical family. After training at Bart's she became a ward sister at the Royal Free under Mr James Berry and when he took his surgical unit out to Serbia and Montenegro in 1915 he asked that she should accompany him, especially since she had nursed for nine months in Bulgaria during the Balkan war of 1912-13 and could speak a little Serbian. However she was by then working at a military hospital and we read: 'The War Office showed no disposition to release her. But eventually, insistence on the need of Serbia and of her special fitness for the task, with intercession from high quarters, produced the desired effect'. So off she went to Skopolje and the terrible typhus epidemic, and in due course was appointed Matron to the Anglo-Russian Hospital. Like many of the other staff, both nursing and medical, her health suffered in the appalling Russian climate and she was plagued by rheumatism. In early 1917 this necessitated her repatriation, a fate which she accepted most indignantly at the hands of Lady Muriel. She was awarded the Royal Red Cross medal and unquestionably earned it.

I have mentioned the yellowing flimsy sheets of paper on which the staff of the hospital are recorded. The list includes the names of 64

[2] Mr A. Irvine Robertson, to whom I am most grateful for this information. Following the war, his aunt became Matron of the Deaconess Hospital Edinburgh, and of Princess Louise Kensington, Hospital for Children. During the Blitz of 1940-42 she worked in the Underground stations in London. She died in 1959 aged 80.

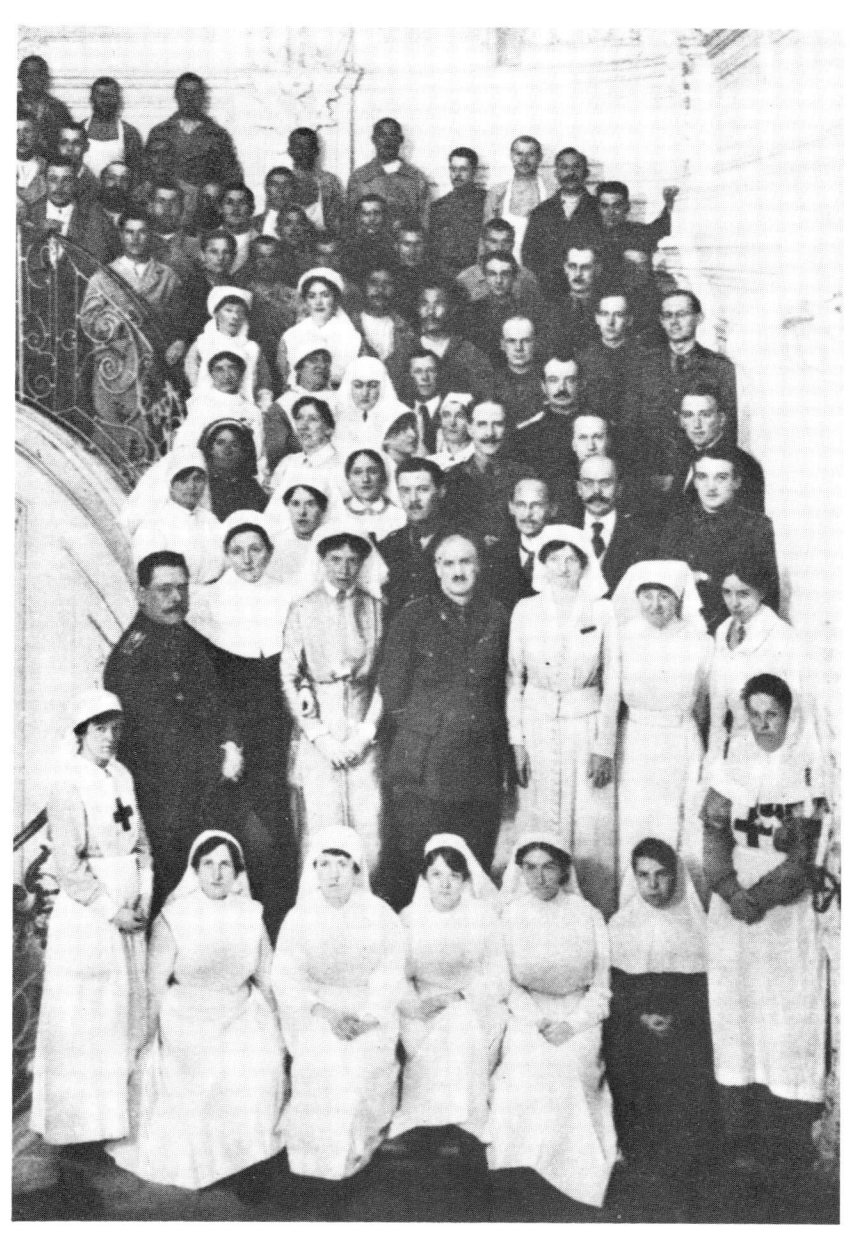

THE GREAT STAIRCASE

51

nurses and VAD's. Among these are a few who have left their mark. I only wish there were more about whom I might write.

One such was Miss Mary MacDonald, one of the senior ward sisters at the Dmitri Palace Hospital. We see her several times in her photograph album, which is inscribed 'Memories of Russia during the War' and which was later presented to the BRCS by her friend Christine Crawford. This album is of more than passing interest because from Miss MacDonald's snapshots were made the dozen photogravure postcards which were sold in very large numbers in aid of the Hospital and three of which are reproduced in this Essay. She was not only in Petrograd and with two of the Field Hospitals but also accompanied Lady Muriel at the time when the rump of the Mobile Unit had to be evacuated from the Southern Front through Odessa and thence by the Trans-Siberian Railway to Vladivostock, Japan and the USA before they reached haven in England in May 1918. Of all the sisters Miss MacDonald may well have had the worst time but for a biographer she is of inestimable value. Amongst her photographs is one of the hideous Army barracks at Lutsk in which Mr Jefferson did splendid work (and there is a group in which he almost certainly features); there are several of Lady Muriel, though none of Lady Sybil; there is one of Mr Thompson and the young Alexis Homiakov who strove so valiantly, presumbly with Miss MacDonald's help, at Kirli-Baba in the Carpathians. Horsedrawn ambulance carts appear alongside a faded print of a Red Cross Daimler which could grace the Veteran Car Rally any year. There is a fuzzy picture labelled 'X-Ray Room', which may or may not have pleased Dr Flavelle, but which should surely find a place in the library of the Faculty of Radiologists. This is the stuff of History.

There was also 'Miss S', the VAD who took tea with the Tsarina to the chagrin of Lady Georgina. Having already done splendid work in France she felt justified in making her own views known concerning the management of the hospital:

> The rubs of the place are now appearing. It wants a real man at the head instead of two very delightful women who move by their own impulses. They are both (the Matron and Lady MP) still at the field station so I haven't seen them. Everyone likes them but they evidently haven't enough strength . . .

She takes a possibly justifiable swipe at the trained nurses, who tended to look down on VAD's:

In fact I don't see why they grumble, but they do, mostly I think because they imagined that they were going out to tea every day and the Russians have other things to do.

Oh my paws and whiskers! One should not takes sides of course but Blunt adds that Miss S. was a considerable social success and proof enough that the Russians had plenty of leisure when they so wished.

A few other names appear in the records. Miss Mildred Mitchener, described on her Red Cross Identity Card as an Anglo-Russian nun, worked as an orderly in the hospital. In the Staircase photograph several women in nun's veils may be seen. Perhaps she is amongst them. We read also of Miss McLeod and Countess Olga and WDH's diary mentions Sisters Farrar, Adcock, Lewis and Kerr. There were many others of course but two unnamed ladies are worthy of record, escorting a group of patients from Galatz, the base hospital of one of the famous Dr Elsie Inglis's Scottish Women's Hospitals which she had established in Serbia, Roumania and South Russia. WDH's diary contains this factual statement: 'Some patients, one blind, arrived from Scottish Women's Hospital to-day'. Lady Sybil seems to have taken more note of their escorts:

> One I *supposed* was a woman and the other I literally thought was a man or at least a fat boy. They are all suffragettes, but it is *quite* unnecessary for them to look as they do. The girl was a chauffeur of an ambulance; she had on a cowboy hat . . . a huge khaki overcoat with a Tommy's haversack on her back and puttees and boots. The overcoat, which made her look *yards* broad, had tartan shoulder-straps with silver thistles. She stood with her legs a yard apart and both hands in her pockets; and I wondered why a straw wasn't hanging out of one corner of her mouth.

Poor Lady Sybil: she preferred the starched white apron with the Red Cross on its bosom.

The fact is that there were an astonishing number of individuals, enthusiasts and philanthropists, men and women, milling about on the Eastern Front in those years, doing their bit to help. For instance the Royal Automobile Club held a meeting and several members 'put themselves, their cars *and their chauffeurs* [my italics] at the disposal of the Red Cross'. Commander Locker-Lampson, the racing motorist, raised a couple of armoured cars and so on.

How the Russians kept track of them all I do not know but it seems that almost anyone was welcome to help since their own facilities were unable to cope with the huge number of casualties. In any case the general direction of the war effort was beginning to crack during 1916 and in 1917 became almost non-existent. Initially it had been very good indeed, being based on an organisation of a character unknown in other countries. This was the Union of Zemstvos and it complemented the work of the Army Medical Services and the Russian Red Cross. The Zemstvos corresponded roughly to our County Councils and from local taxes were able to set up refugee centres, canteens, disinfecting units, bacteriological laboratories and vaccination clinics etc. As the war progressed they established their own hospitals, undertook the transport of medical stores, repaired ambulances and even roads and bridges. An all-embracing organisation indeed.

The Russian Red Cross itself was most highly organised and demanded the highest standards in its recruitment of nurses. I cannot do better in closing this chapter than record Miss Farmborough's own account of her initiation as a *Krestovaya Sestra*.

Before each jewelled icon the *lampada* glowed with a ruby light. On each High Altar the high brass candlesticks held steadily shining candles; near them stood a silver chalice containing Holy Water, with the Book of Books alongside. A priest in full canonicals entered & made his way towards the altar. Soon his rich, resonant voice was heard reciting the beautiful Slavonik prayers of the Greek Orthodox liturgy. Heads were reverently bowed. The censer was swung to & fro, emitting trembling breaths of fine grey fragrant smoke. Finally there was silence.

The golden-robed priest rose from his knees, crucifix in hand, faced the congregation. The nurses moved in relays to kneel at the altar. Over each he intoned a prayer, placed the red cross on her white apron and held the crucifix to her lips. Now he was standing before me. 'Your name?' 'Florence'. 'Of the *pravoslavsny* [orthodox] church?' 'No, of the Church of England'. A whispered consultation, the book was referred to. I was cold with fear. Then, the prescribed ritual, his tongue twisting at the foreign name: 'To thee, Floronz, child of God, servant of the Most High, is given this token of faith, of home, of charity. With faith shalt thou follow Christ the Master, with hope shalt thou look towards Christ for thy salvation, with charity shalt thou fulfil thy duties. Thou shalt tend the sick, the wounded, the needy: with words of comfort shalt thou cheer them.'

Two years later Miss Farmborough had reason to remember her vow. During the Brusilov offensive on the Southern Front she dealt with many mortally wounded. 'Once, I questioned our head doctor about these injections. "This man is dying: he is already in a coma. If I inject camphor or caffeine, he will only revive to feel intense pain. Shall I leave him to die in peace?" He glared at me and his wrathful voice made answer: "Sister Florence, do your duty! What right have you to dispute orders? Have you forgotten the supreme duty of Red Cross work: to do everything in one's power to preserve and restore life?" I knew that he was right: he always was.'

Petrograd: Marking Time

It had always been understood by the London Committee and the Foreign Office that the hospital should be an entirely self-supporting unit, only the accommodation being provided by the Russians. The original plan had been for the despatch of a Field Hospital directly to the Front but Sir George Buchanan had wisely vetoed this, realising that some sort of Base Hospital would be essential. Lady Muriel's reply was to suggest a hospital of 400 beds in Petrograd, to be fed by three field hospitals. Nothing of this sort was available and in any case the Russians had enough beds of their own to cope with the casualties from their North-Western Front, which at that time of the year was largely static.

Lady Sybil and her advance guard had received a 'red carpet' reception when they arrived (as she wrote) 'after a capital journey'. But they found little else to cheer them. Petrograd was bursting at its seams. More than half a million refugees had descended on the city; everything was in short supply and the Russian doctors had their hands full of their own problems. Therefore she had to set about looking for accommodation and in the process they were taken to see several hospitals in the City by the Mayor, Count Tolstoy. Lady Sybil's account of 6th October gives some details:

> Saw one big hospital of 680 beds in one room. Used to be a shed where all the tram-cars were kept at night. Most of the theatre sisters who work here are society ladies and wear big pearl ear-rings and quality rings.
>
> We were taken to see the Dental Hosp. where 90 wounded lie with broken jaws, blown-off noses etc. The Hosp. itself was filthy but the surgery quite excellent, most ingenious and clever. It is wonderful to see how they build up chins, noses etc. out of nothing . . . intensely interesting but many very horrible sights.

She was amazed at the number of women doctors. 'How unlike England: sometimes the Chief Surgeon is a woman and the Second a man.' She was delighted to meet a Mrs Chambers, an English nurse who had been on a hospital train for four months, usually carrying about 500 wounded at each trip. 'Normally four Sisters on the train but two are ill of enteric, so now there is only herself and another, neither having had any real training. There are two surgeons on the train. One is very good; the other is very bad, having lost his nerve. He is really a physician and trembles if he has to operate which, alas! he has to do only too often and even the orderlies can hardly bear to see him work.' Alas! indeed; but such experiences made her the more determined to do better for her own hospital.

Other hospitals were visited as well. (There were said to be several hundred in Petrograd and 1,275 in Moscow.) One such was the Winter Palace Hospital itself, to which Ian Malcolm and Lady Sybil had been invited for the opening ceremony: 'the only foreigners there; not a diplomat, nobody but Russians of the Court, all in gorgeous uniforms and strung all over with medals and orders like an Xmas tree'. They were not too impressed by the hospital itself, since the wards had been converted from the huge State Rooms and '100 beds in one ward is really too big'. On the other hand the organisation of the ceremony impressed them tremendously and Lady Sybil wrote enthusiastically about the priests in their green and gold vestments and the Imperial Choir, 'in claret red and gold, singing the Graces'.

Afterwards, to another small 50-bedded hospital — 'the only one I have seen where the men, every single one of them, smiled and looked happy. I must try and get that atmosphere into our hospital'. Thus, Lady Sybil. But then: 'Yesterday afternoon I went over the saddest place, the big central hospital for limbless soldiers . . . Somehow when you saw these great numbers of legless men it makes your heart ache for all this wrecked humanity. Far the saddest sight were the men with absolutely no legs at all, just trunks — great big men cut off in the middle. If they were standing on the ground they came up to one's elbow'.

A week later, a further extract from her diary:

> Still going over hospitals. One beautiful one to-day, the Head Surgeon being the doctor that looked after the Czarevitch. He told us that there now over twenty thousand men in Russia who have lost their arms or legs. Yesterday we motored eighty miles through snow and slush with Prof. Sherkoovenko who wished to show us some hospitals in the country. We saw Mr.

Fabergé's house where he has wounded officers, about twenty in one part of the house: the rest is a museum of every conceivable thing, jade, miniatures, books, stamps, etc.

After this unique visit to the Aladdin's Cave of the world's greatest jeweller (who died in exile in Switzerland following the Revolution), Lady Sybil 'looked across the water to the Fortress of Kronstadt about 20 miles away with the sun setting in a golden glory'. Then back to Petrograd to meet for the first time, the Grand Duke Dmitri who was to play such a large part in her life and in that of the Hospital. 'A very nice boy', she noted.

Reading these jottings now, I feel again the urge of her humanity.

Within no time at all Lady Sybil sent off her first report to Lord Cheylesmore:

> The Petrograd Committee have the honour to report the following to the Executive Committee in London:
>   Mr. Poluvtzoff, one of the Heads of the Russian Red Cross for the Petrograd District, who whilst expressing satisfaction of the Russian Red X at the arrival of a hospital Unit from Great Britain, informed us we must understand that with the best will in the world considerable difficulty would be found in housing the Hospital adequately, owing to all the best buildings having been already taken. Altogether three buildings have been visited.

One was the Stroganov Palace but was discarded as too small; another might have done but 'it was badly situated in a back street and was unsuitable in other minor ways'. [This was in fact the German Embassy. They were advised that the Russian soldiers were so superstitious that, had they been admitted to such a place, they would have assumed that they were being sent there to die.] The third was the Palace of the Grand Duke Dmitri.

Two days later she made this simple record in her diary: *Grand Duke Dmitri offers his Palace.* Obviously there must have been a lot of diplomatic activity behind the scenes and it was the Ambassador, Sir George Buchanan, who had clinched the deal. The Grand Duke himself — 'a nice attractive-looking boy but somewhat dissipated', was Lady Sybil's second assessment — had apparently not been too happy in his inheritance, which had been given to him by his aunt the Grand Duchess Serge, a sister of the Tsarina. His butler had recently hanged himself in the Palace and because this event had cast a rather

58

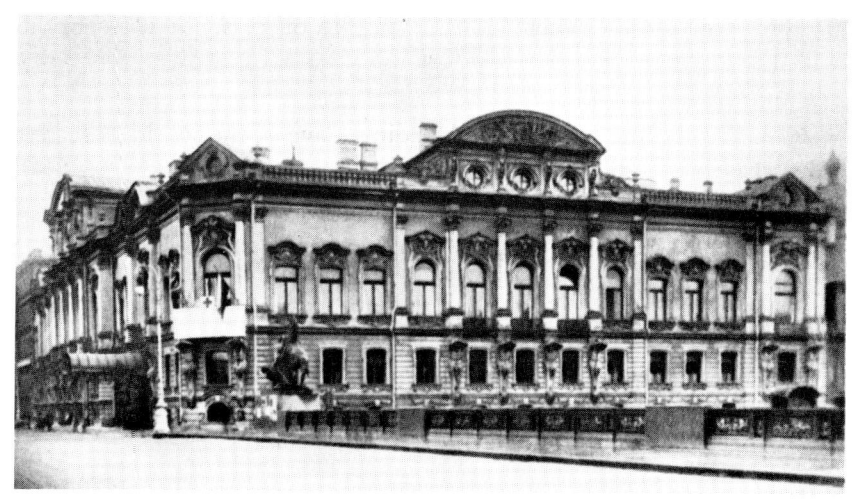

THE DMITRI PALACE

ugly spell on the house he was happy to see it turned over for a useful and benevolent function, provided he could continue to live in a part of it. This he did when he was not at the Front, though with results which could have hardly been foreseen at the time and which had a profound effect on the hospital eighteen months later. His personal apartments were on the ground floor and one entrance to them was a door near to the foot of the great staircase which features in one of my illustrations. Moreover the attics of the Palace continued to be occupied by 'a swarm of old family retainers', which must indeed have added to the complications of converting it into a hospital.

The Palace[1] itself was a superb building and its situation on the Nevsky Prospekt, one of the finest boulevards in the whole of Europe, could hardly have been bettered. Dr Fleming, inspecting it for the first time, was less than pleased; and justifiably, since it had virtually no plumbing: but he accepted that beggars could not be choosers and so in the harsh winter of 1915, which seems to have descended like an Iron Curtain, they set about organising a 200-bedded hospital.

[1] I refer to it in my account as the Dmitri Palace and it was thus known to the Committee and Staff of the A-R H. To the Russians it remained the Sergei Palace, after its former owner.

Plumbing, baths and so on were installed. The damask walls of the *piano nobile* were boarded up, the parquet flooring covered with linoleum; only the chandeliers remained; but 'all this will lead to considerable expense. The estimates are being got ready, it is difficult to say what they are likely to be'.

Lady Sybil was in her element. 'Hours of plans and measurements. Have to accept as the best thing possible. It is a fine Palace and we will fly two big Union Jacks over it!' She bullied her architect — 'a little dwarf three feet high' — and quite unjustly it would seem, since he was giving his services free and all materials were in the shortest supply. And when the estimates did come in she was able to report that the alterations would cost one to two thousand pounds and would take about six weeks to do. She also added a familiar phrase, 'Labour difficult'. Heavens above! Two thousand pounds and six weeks for converting a Palace into a hospital, with labour problems to boot: the mind boggles . . . Well, she got it done.

Having lost all their equipment they had to go shopping. How they acquired 200 bedsteads and mattresses is not on record but WDH recounted one example of Russian business acumen. 'The Matron asked the price of a sink for the theatre an was told 75 roubles. When she said it was for the Anglo-Russian Hospital the manager of the store said he had made a mistake and it was 175 roubles.' It will be recalled that amongst the supplies which were immured in the arctic ice were the hospital's X-ray machines and on his arrival WDH was asked to advise about their replacement. On the back of Lady Sybil's Report and written in pencil in his own hand, I find this astonishing recommendation, astonishing at least to anyone familiar with the contemporary cost of radiological apparatus:

> After consulting with Dr Flavelle I have the honour to report that I think,
>
> (1) that a sum of £60 — £70 should be spent on the purchase of additional apparatus: Chemicals (i.e. about £38) and some small instruments which Dr Flavelle regards as urgently required.
>
> (2) that later on a more elaborate outfit may be necessary, in which case the details of the apparatus required can be forwarded to England. Such an outfit, if it is composed of the very best materials, as supplied by Messrs Butt & Co., will cost the hospital between £300 & £400.

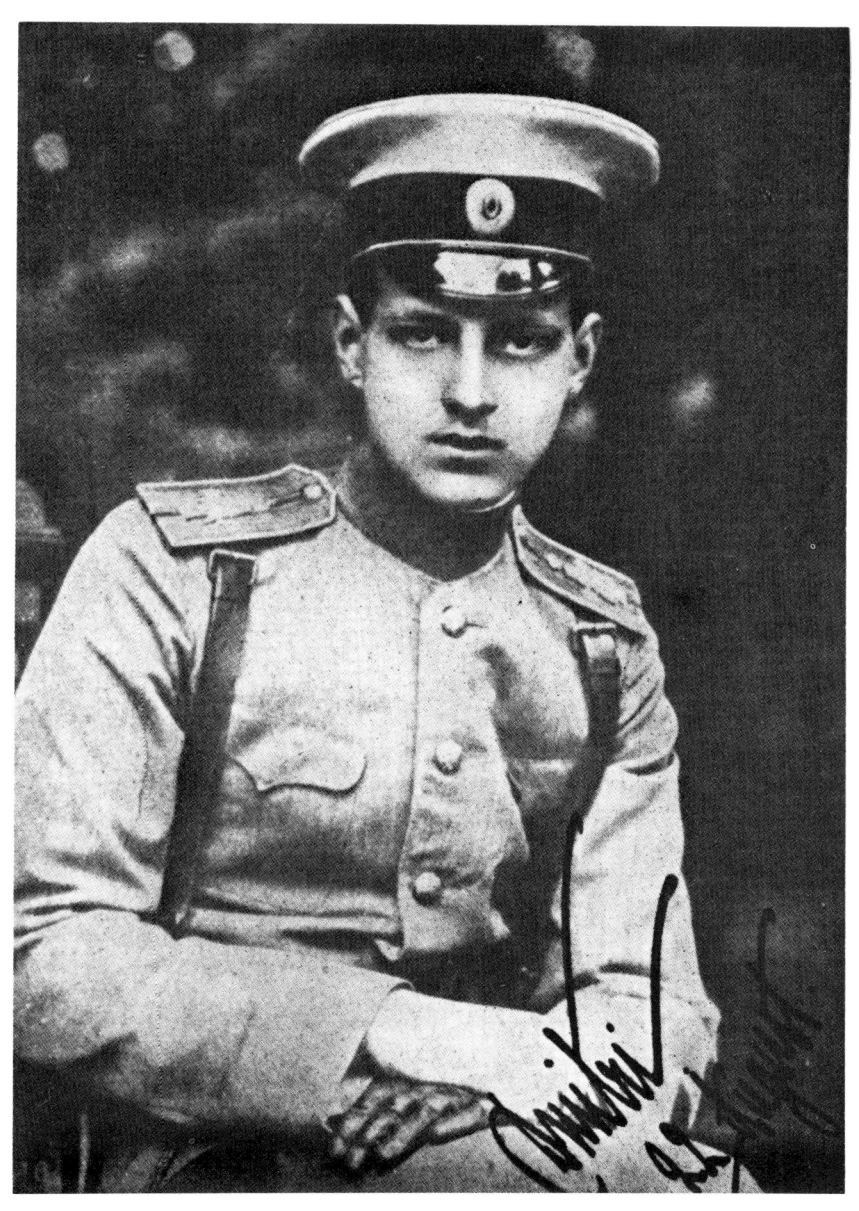

THE GRAND DUKE DMITRI PAVLOVICH

The political side of the Hospital could not be neglected. Within ten days of their arrival Lady Sybil and Mr Ian Malcolm MP were bidden to attend the Tsarina at Tsarskoe Selo, the Summer Palace, which was half an hour by train from Petrograd. They were received by flunkies, one more glorious than another and walked through room upon room 'until we came to where a Lady-in-Waiting was waiting for us; a very small and gay little thing who said the Empress would soon be disengaged. Almost immediately an old Lady, very like the old Duchess of Buccleuch, dressed in violet with a housekeeper's cap upon her exalted head and covered with diamond orders, waddled into the room. She was the Mistress of the Court. I . . . was led away by the Major Domo, a gentleman with the most marvellous headgear I have ever seen. He wore a tightly-fitting cap of red and gold embroidery with a small feather of red over one ear, and over the other a round thing of some gorgeous stuff of many colours and then two huge ostrich feathers of orange, white and black'. He conducted Lady Sybil to the Empress's door where she was taken over by 'a coal-black slave (sic) with a turban and beautiful clothes and in I went'. After this impressive prelude the Tsarina was almost an anti-climax. She was dressed as a nurse. 'It suited her extra-ordinarily well and she looked very, very handsome. I had envisaged a cold tragic face with all life gone out of it. Instead of this it was a beautiful face, full of sympathy and charm.' They talked for 20 minutes or so and Lady Sybil came away feeling that she had never before experienced an atmosphere which cried out for so much sympathy.

Two days later they had a repeat performance with the Dowager Tsarina, so that there can be little doubt that the Anglo-Russian Hospital was having all the stops pulled out for it by the Establishment. She was once again 'guarded by a coal-black gentleman, which seems the fashion for Empresses. She sent many messages to my delightful father [remembering] the most interesting morning she spent with him at Hampstead and of the old actress (Pavlova) that he took to see her there'. [This can scarcely be considered a flattering description of the famous ballerina, who at that time was only 30 years of age and at the height of her fame]. At this time too Lady Sybil recorded that she was 'out every single night in the last ten days and tomorrow the Ballet again. To the Opera to hear Chaliapine with the young Pierre Obolenskys. The Russians are certainly the kindest people'.

The 'social round' continued and here it may be recorded that when Lady Muriel arrived in 1916 she brought all her jewelry with her so that she might appear suitably dressed for the 'Tolstoyan Receptions' which she expected to attend. At the end of the affair she secreted them behind the altar of the English church and there, 13 years later, she found them untouched when she returned to look after her Distressed British Subjects. This fact helped to confirm her belief that the Bolsheviks were not really revolutionaries (even when she was accused by them of spying in 1934) because she had a profound belief in the basic Russian *ethos,* sympathised with the principal of replacing the dictatorship of the Tsar by a democratic government and was unwilling to believe that one tyranny could be replaced by another which proved to be immeasurably worse.

Another example of the evident political importance of the Anglo-Russian Hospital was an invitation to attend the annual Saint George's Day celebration in the People's Palace, the Albert Hall of St Petersburg. Mr Ian Malcolm, the Matron, Dr Fleming and Lady Sybil were the only foreigners present, all the other guests being those who had either been awarded the Cross of St George for bravery in the field or the St George's Medal. Prince Oldenburg, 82 years of age, was in charge of the arrangements, which included the feeding of 16,000 soldiers 'sitting at four-a-and-half kilometres of tables, all with white tablecloths: 8,000 chickens and I forget how many tons of other meats'. Each man had a bottle of red wine to himself and a bottle of wine made from some preparation of honey — 'very potent, I am told'. The entire hall was decorated with the orange and black banners of St George, set against the pure white galleries and pillars of the Opera House. There were three bands in the galleries, the entire chorus from the Opera, a platform for the priests with altar, cross and icon. Red Cross nurses were everywhere, looking after the wounded of whom there were many and all of whom had an orange and black ribbon on his arm-sling or bandaged head or over his heart. After the first course, 12 silver trumpets, each seven feet long, blew a mighty fanfare from the top gallery and then 'the Old Prince called for the Emperor's health. Every soldier rose while the three Bands played the National Anthem accompanied by the Choir and the 12 silver trumpets. The men went on cheering when the Bands stopped, so they recommenced . . . this happened three times and never stopped for a second'.

The junketings went on until 5 a.m. but 'for those who were

wounded and some badly wounded, there was far too much emotion. I have never seen anything better arranged: not a hitch anywhere'. But then Lady Sybil added this: 'It is curious how the Russians can organise a thing so superbly — and yet make such a hopeless fiasco of things that really matter'. My mind goes back to our hotel in Leningrad where my wife and I had been waiting nearly two hours for breakfast in the restaurant and hearing a plaintive American voice from a nearby table saying: 'How these guys got Gagarin into space beats me!'

Easter is the supreme expression of the Orthodox Church and in Tsarist times it must have reached its apogee. In one of his early letters WDH remarked upon the astounding quality of Russian singing when he attended a Cathedral service — 'peasants who are illiterate yet can sing in parts'. He wrote about 'a wonderful concert here in the hospital given by a special choir of deacons from different churches. A curious set of men with strange wild faces and untidy hair hanging down to their shoulders but with marvellous voices. They sang 12 Russian hymns and anthems, ending with a prayer for the Tsar'.

On Good Friday there was a special service in the Dmitri Palace. A coffin with a painted effigy was carried round the wards. The following night WDH attended a midnight service in the Private Chapel of the Ministry of the Grand Dukes. His diary:

> Very long and monotonous. Crowds of men and women in evening dress. Everyone holding a candle. At 12 Priest announced that Christ was risen. Candles extinguished. Kissing, three times all round. Afterwards returned to Hosp. where service cont. till 3 am, when supper arrived. In streets throngs of people and houses lit up — great day in Russia.

(The entry for this day ends on a more secular note: 'Heard about riots in Ireland'.)

Miss Florence Farmborough, far away at the Front, recorded the same event in more dramatic words: 'Into our little church the soldiers streamed cheek by jowl with officers of all ranks. Rank, birth, grade, these did not exist. It was a happy and deeply emotional service. Lighted candles blazed, devout fingers traced the Sign of the Cross. Then came the culmination: *Kristos Voskres* and the triumphant reply: *Voystinu Voskrece* (He is indeed risen). And then the three kisses on brow, on either cheek — evoking God's blessing: the Father, the Son, the Holy Spirit . . . and the time-honoured Easter eggs, painted in brilliant colours'. She also recounted how the priests had to be dissuaded from a candlelight procession along the front trenches, less than a 100 metres from the Germans . . .

Easter being also a time for gifts, WDH went shopping: 'I have been buying you a "prévenant" as I felt I must send you a token for Easter. I think you will like it as it is a special kind of enamel work which they make here. I chose a cigarette case because I thought you would be able to carry it about with you always and you will notice that the enamel is peculiar in being transparent which makes it all the more interesting and beautiful. It was not really expensive — only R.30 — and so you need not think that I was extravagant'. He also bought 'a good painted Ikon in the Jews' Market' for seven roubles. The cigarette-case lies on my desk as I write these words, while on the painted icon, Metrophan first Archbishop of Voronezh, looks down on me from a nearby wall, raising his right hand in blessing as he does so. At seven roubles to the pound, the former cost about £4, the latter £1. In 1964 an icon expert valued this for me at about £50 adding that 'Christ or Mary would have been worth more', an opinion with which Mrs Talbot-Rice emphatically disagrees — on artistic grounds I should add.

While the hospital was being prepared, Lady Sybil had problems with her staff. 'High time the hospital opened as a lot of nurses without work are very childish and unreasonable', she wrote to her mother. Nor did the doctors fare much better because we have the testimony of a Mrs Ethel Lindley, also writing to Countess Grey with news of her daughter: '[Sybil] is perfectly marvellous at keeping everything going and I am beginning to realise what terribly kittle cattle Doctors & nurses are, particularly doctors! They seem so incapable of seeing anyone's point of view & the Russian point of view is not easy to see in any case . . .'

Everyone put in time at the Berlitz School but they found Russian a very difficult language to master. Lady Muriel did her best to learn it *in absentia* but Lady Sybil clearly loathed it: 'all my spare time is spent trying to learn this foul language. My head is split at all the different endings of the different verbs. I . . . walk about with horrid little bits of paper that have countless words on them to learn'. WDH despaired: 'I don't think I'll ever manage to speak it — or understand it', he wrote home.

There were other things to do though. Mark Gardner went off to Archangel to see if the stores from the *Abaris*[2] could be located and off-loaded. He returned empty handed. Fleming went down to Kiev to investigate the possibility of setting up a field hospital, and later he and WDH visited Helsingfors to negotiate the purchase of ambulance carts. They reported that they could obtain 33 carts for 13,000 Roubles which struck WDH as reasonable, but the deal fell through. Gould May and Jones went to Moscow to try and buy equipment. None was available. Perhaps the Commandant himself should have gone because their visit provoked WDH to write in his diary:

> Fleming seems inclined to sit down in P. & it seems doubtful whether he is playing the game entirely. Have just seen Pares who is a wild enthusiast & seems to have the confidence of the people at the front though he is not popular here & is considered a madman. Fleming obviously dislikes him. [He obviously did, because a week later there is this entry:]
> Pares dined in mess & was treated by Fleming in an insulting & irritating manner.

It seems plain that tensions were rising at this time and that here was the beginning of the 'near-mutiny' mentioned in an earlier chapter and which Lady Sybil was reluctantly forced to suppress. And this is supported by some further entries in the diary too: 'May has been doing some very plain speaking the last 2 days & his remarks have been taken better than one might expect. May & Flavelle v. dissatisfied'.

There were also some quite considerable health problems. Waterhouse went down with a carbuncle. WDH had a miserable time with an inner-ear infection which plagued him for several weeks and eventually led to him having a radical mastoidectomy. Miss Irvine Robertson was ill and many of the nurses were laid up: 'they simply will not listen to reason or understand that it is a very cold country and a vile climate'. At one time or another everyone succumbed; Lady Sybil developed mumps ('of all ridiculous things'), Lady Muriel typhoid fever, which was far worse of course. At least none of them died!

The cold that winter was to them quite unbelievable, the wind piercing. Lady Sybil welcomed the snow when it came, not least

---

[2] There must have been another supply ship as well since WDH makes several references to the *Mereddio* in his letters.

because it would hold up the fighting, but she observed that 'the sun doesn't shine like in Canada'. All the letters, reports and diaries of this time were full of it. 'If people like us rarely get our rooms above 50°, what must it be for the poor?' 'Terrible cold again; between 20° and 30° below zero. How do the men in the trenches survive?' And so on.[3] Yet there were some compensations: 'St Isaac's Cathedral next door, lately completely covered with snow is quite beautiful, pillars and all looking like white alabaster, bronze statues against the white, the whole surmounted with a golden dome. The two lovely slender graceful gold spires take every glimpse of sunshine one ever gets'.

When the hospital was eventually ready the VIPs came to inspect it. The Ambassador declared himself enchanted with it. The Grand Duchess Serge announced that she would be there at 8.15 in the morning, coming from Tsarskoe Selo, and so Lady Sybil and Dr Fleming drove from the Club, where they were staying at the time, at 7.45 a.m. 'with the thermometer registering 30° below zero and Dr. F. assuring me that he would soon become an anarchist' in order to receive her; only to find that she had already been there for half an hour. It was the Grand Duchess who suggested that Lady Sybil and the Matron should live in. 'She is very good looking and is called the German Madonna: very unpopular now in Moscow instead of idolised as before.' According to WDH both she and the Dowager Tsarina looked exactly like Queen Alexandra, 'at any rate from behind'.

WDH expressed pained surprise that no important Russian doctors came to visit the hospital, which seems to confirm once again that the establishment of the hospital was basically a political move. About this time he wrote to my mother:

> Our hospital is full of septic wounds: sooner or later they all pour pus. We have to work incessantly with continuous carifation [? scarification] etc. to keep them going. It is also very difficult to ventilate properly in this climate. It is so cold that you simply can't open windows for more than a few minutes at a

[3] The Réaumur scale was used in Russia at this time. Fahrenheit (1710) had proposed a scale from 32° (freezing) to 212° (boiling): Réaumur (1730) from 0° to 80°: Celsius (1742) from 0° to 100°, now generally known as Centigrade. The difficulty arises in trying to calculate the 'degrees of frost below zero'. At any rate it was extremely cold: as also was the winter of 1916-17.

time. Result, the wounds all smell and before we know what has happened we get temperatures flying about and all kinds of indefinite fevers. I only hope we shan't get erysipelas or something worse.

I don't think we are very popular. The medical profession here have given us the cold shoulder: none of their well-known men has come near us . . . one can't mistake the meaning of it.

In *The Work of the Anglo-Russian Hospital* there is a full account of the hospital at the time of its commission:

The hospital, as completed, had accommodation for a hundred and eighty-eight beds, and these at a pinch could be increased to two hundred. The Concert Hall with the two large reception rooms all opening on each other, constituted the three main wards. These rooms, large, light and lofty, with great windows going up to the ceiling, made ideal wards and gave accommodation for 150 beds without overcrowding. Opening out of them or in close proximity were a linen and duty room, bath room, lavatories, and a large dressing room with four tables and with hot and cold water laid on, where all the daily dressings were done, as is the custom on the Continent. Beyond the dressing room, and with an entrance opposite the main staircase, was the patients' dining room, and beyond this again three smaller wards which contained the balance of the beds. The operating theatre with adjoining anaesthetic and sterilising rooms, the X-ray department and the bacteriological laboratory were on the same floor but in an isolated part of the building. A large room beyond the laboratory was partitioned into three for two of the surgeons and the two dressers, who always slept on the premises. The offices were, perhaps, the worst feature of the whole building, being cramped and inconvenient. A part of the passage adjoining the chapel and between the theatre and the last small ward was set aside for the dentist and his outfit. On the ground floor to the right of the main entrance was the dispensary, and in the basement were the kitchens where also provision was made for a carpenter's shop and a store room for soiled linen.

The arrangements, generally, made for the maximum of efficiency, but one of the greatest difficulties was the lack of storage accommodation.

Two days before the hospital was officially opened a superb silver-gilt icon was presented to the Committee of the Hospital by 'a group of Russian friends'. A plate on the back of the case proclaims (with a charming mis-spelling which is singularly appropriate):

> *To the Comity of Anglo-Russian Hospital as a memento from his Russian friends.*
> *V. N. Shenkumenko. N. Melnikov. Prince P. Obolenski.*
> *A. Fenz. Tikchev. A. Polontzev.*
> *Count A. C. Musiu-Pushkin.*
>
> *Petrograd 12 January 1916*

The icon was painted and the case made by the monks of an unknown Monastery, probably in the early XIXth Century. It depicts Saint Ouar, Martyr who is commemorated on 19th October together with seven teachers of Christianity, Saint Cleopatra and her son. Ouar was a soldier during the reign of the Emperor Maximan. He died strung from a tree *circa* 307 AD and his seven teachers were beheaded shortly afterwards (hence his martyrdom). Saint Cleopatra, a holy widow from Palestine, took his relics there and founded a church in his name. Her son John died on the day of the consecration of the new church and Cleopatra saw both her son and Ouar in a vision (hence his sanctification). She herself died peacefully in 327 AD.

After the painting of the icon was completed the case was sealed and only the head and hands of the martyr and above these the head of the Deity, would have been visible. After the war, the icon was presented to the British Red Cross Society by Lady Sybil Middleton (as she had then become) and it stands today in the Small Board Room of their Headquarters in Grosvenor Crescent, London. But with a difference. The Case has been opened and hinged and the painting restored so that, after 150 years or so, the skill of the monk who painted it may once again be observed.[4]

---

[4] The restoration and renovation was done in 1969 by Mr David Montravelli, a native of Georgia, who pointed out that such paintings were done on a gelatin base which makes them extremely delicate and difficult to clean. The restoration was a personal gift to the BRCS by Mrs C. F. Fawcett, Archivist to the Society. The distinguished historian of Russian Art, Mrs Tamara Talbot-Rice is of the opinion that the case is a finer example of icon work than the painting itself. This view is shared by Mr John Stuart of Sotheby's who considers the case to be of Dutch design and who discovered the history of the Sainted Martyr on my behalf.

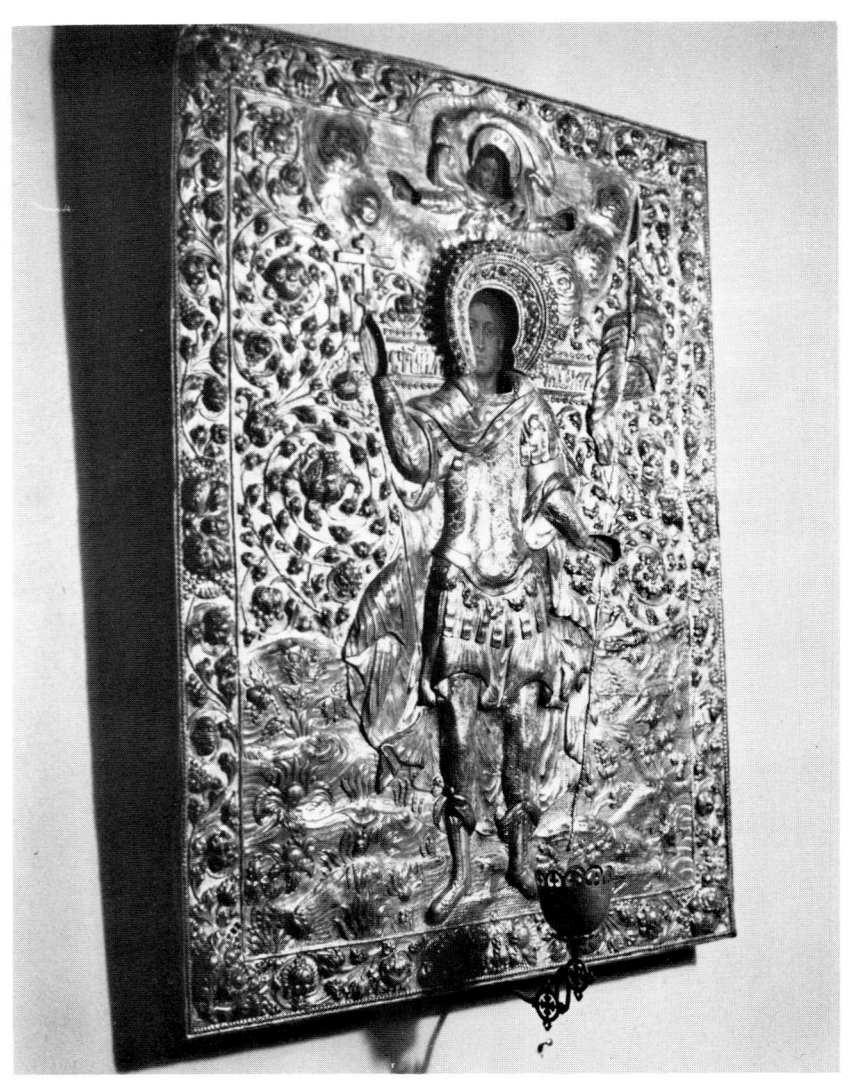

THE ICON CLOSED

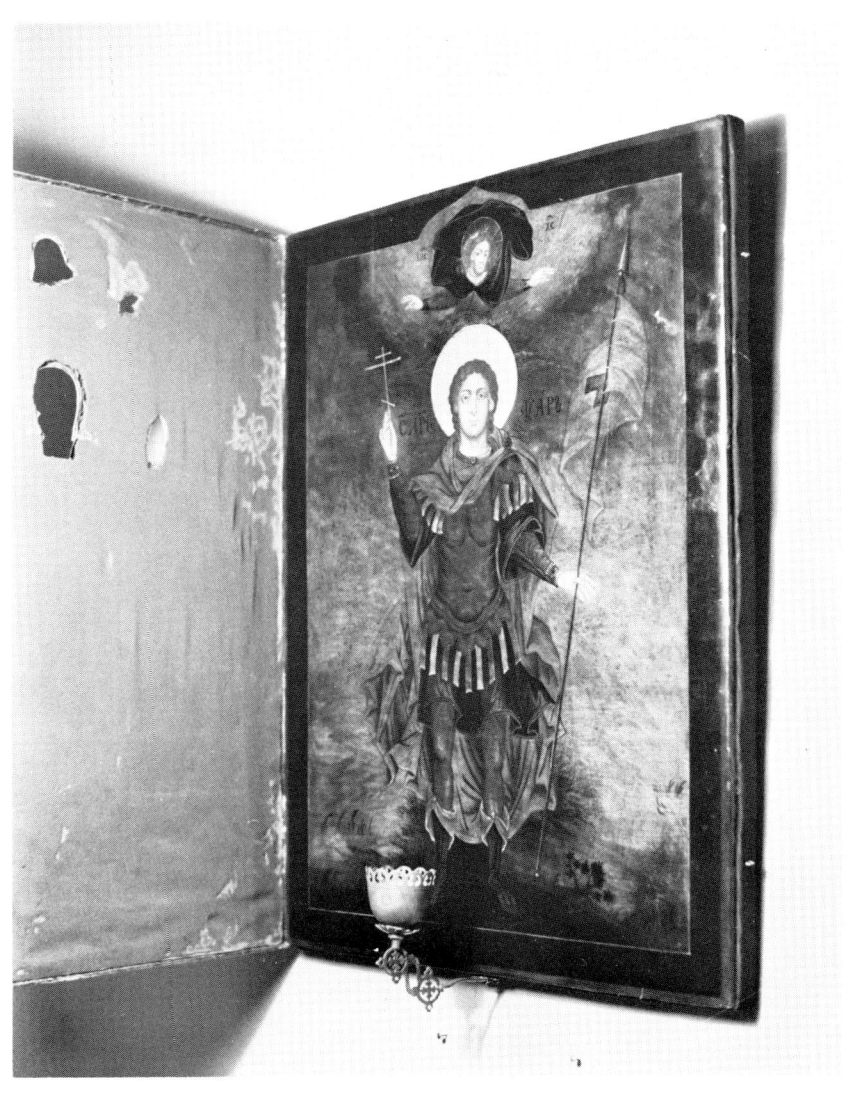

THE ICON OPENED

The opening ceremony took place on 18th January 1916 (OS) or 31st January (English date) according to the published Report. It was a grand affair but like everything else connected with the hospital, it raised its own problems. The Grand Duke claimed the right to make the arrangements: after all it was his Palace. And his aunt, the Grand Duchess Serge who had given it to him, would have liked to have opened it herself. But she willingly agreed to stand down in favour of the Tsarina who had been invited to do so by Dmitri and who had accepted. However as Lady Sybil observed: 'of course we will have to have the Dowager Empress as well. It will give us a good shove off!' For of course she was the Patroness of the hospital. The Embassy demurred; it would be impossible to have both of them because of doubts about precedence. At this point it is necessary to explain that, unlike Great Britain, which between 1952 and 1953 had three living Queens (two of whom accepted that they took less precedence than the Queen Regnant Elizabeth II) in Russia it had never been constitutionally decided whether the reigning Tsarina or the widow of the previous Tsar should be the First Lady of the land. It may seem odd that this mattered at all, but such was the case; so a compromise was reached and the Third Lady, the Grand Duchess Vladimir, was invited to perform the necessary functions. She too accepted. Even that wasn't the end of it, for the Dowager Empress, who had been laid low with lumbago, suddenly decided that she would like to officiate and the ceremony had to be put off for a couple of days in order to accommodate her wishes; and (wrote Blunt) 'it needed all Sir George's patience and diplomacy to appease Vladimir'.

In the event all three were present, an almost unique occurrence and one which was regarded as a triumph for Anglo-Russian *entente*. The Tsarina brought her two eldest daughters, Olga and Tatiana, and there were four (or possibly five) other Grand Duchesses and two Grand Dukes, one of whom was Cyril and who later became the Head of the Romanov family. There was of course the Ambassador and Lady Georgina and a host of officers covered with medals and decorations. It must have been a splendid sight for WDH described it, together with a little sketch in his diary, to show where they all stood in the Concert Hall of the Palace:

> Opening of Hospital by Dowager Empress. Staff of Sisters and doctors on left of room. Choir 6 men 10 boys in black uniform with gold braid facings side of altar. Priest with jewelled hat, 2 men with velvet caps & 4 other officers all in golden gowns.

Amused to see them colmbing *(sic)* their hair, one of them with marcelle waving at the back.

Empress arrived punctually in plain black dress with old furs & hat. Seemed diminutive and shrivelled up. Behind her chair two Grand Ds. and two daughters. Eldest dressed well in white, white fur hat & dress: young active face, vivacious with mischievous eyes: distinctly attractive girl.[5]

Service mostly in Russian but some prayers in English for Royal Family & success of allies. Excellent singing. Doctors & nurses knelt while Priest was praying for them. Cross kissed by Empress & retinue. Water sprinkled on crowd with large brush. Procession round wards, theatre etc. headed by priests, then by Empress & officers. Empress chatted with doctors & nurses in each department. Told Thompson he looked very young. 'What, me? said T-', which amused her immensely!

And after all this, nothing! Nothing at all happened for ten days. The beautiful wards, with their chandeliers and potted palms, remained empty and one can imagine the frustration. Mr Bruce, of the British Embassy, was obviously very unhappy and wished to send home a report indicating that the hospital was not proving its value. He told WDH that Sweden was behaving badly and was holding up 150,000 parcels destined for Russia. 'Considerable friction with A', we read. 'A' must have been (Andrew) Fleming, I think, because the next entry reads: 'Fleming & Flavelle have threatened to resign if Committee insist on sending out Bruce's diatribe'. Then there is a story that Lady Muriel, at Fleming's request, had written to Mr Asquith to ask him to persuade 'X' to come out to Petrograd to see things for himself: and that 'X' had replied: 'when *my* Prime Minister asks me to go I cannot possibly refuse'. [Who was 'X'? I do not know.]

On 11th February the first convoy arrived. Morale improved: 'A busy week — mostly medical cases'. By the 17th there were 110 patients in the beds and surgical work began. For the first time in over

[5] This was surely Princess Olga, then 21 years old. Alas, poor Olga! destined to be murdered by the Bolsheviks, with the Tsar and other members of his family, on 16th July 1918 at Ekaterinburg. In the *Gulag Archipelago* Solzhenitsyn writes that P. L. Voikov, Urals Provincial Commissar of Foodstuffs, directed the dismemberment of the corpses, the cremation of the remains and the dispersal of the ashes so that no trace of the Royal Family should remain. Voikov became Ambassador to Poland and was assassinated in Warsaw in 1927.

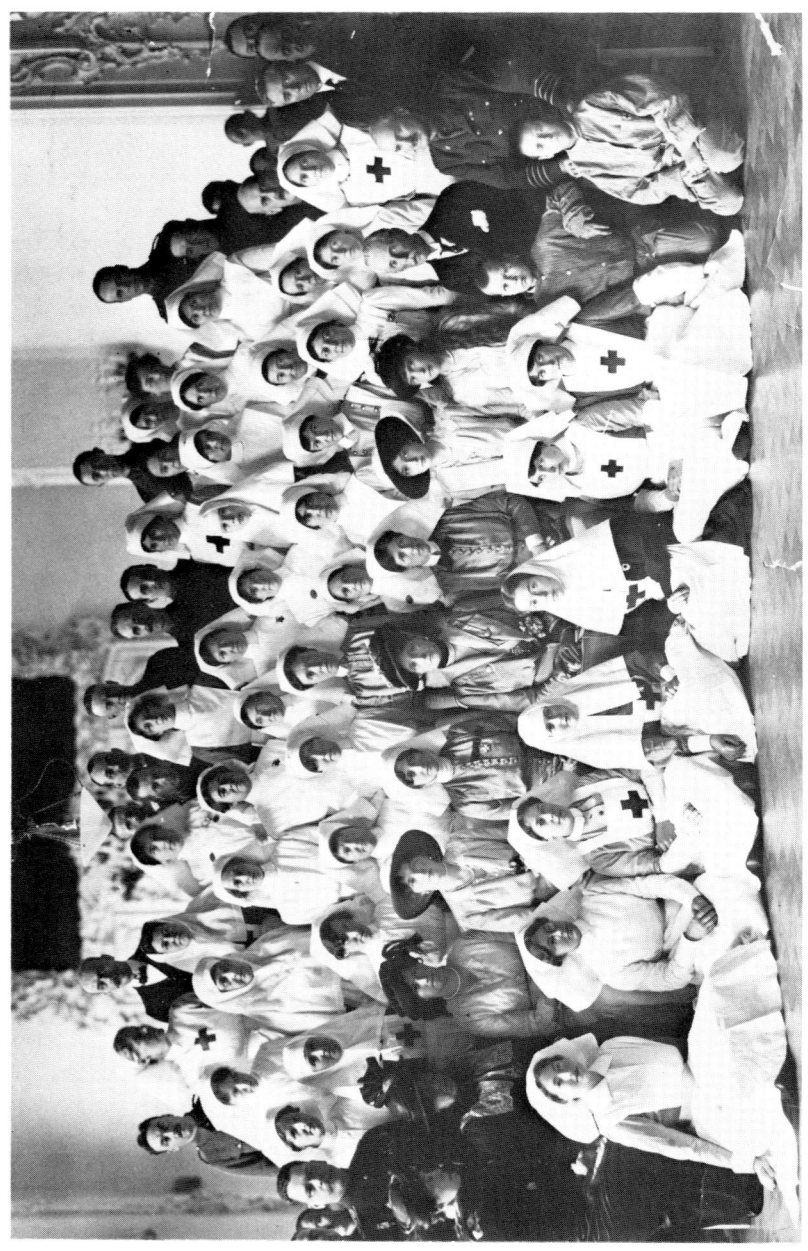

THE TSARINA AND HER FOUR DAUGHTERS

three months WDH was able to wield his scalpel. 'Many wounded by hand grenades, five or six cleaning revolvers — ? accidentally', he noted: which seems to bear out what Lady Muriel was to comment upon the following year and which I mention in a later chapter. Things progressed reasonably well for the next two months though on 31st March there was 'a violent debate re management. Interview with CO, Lady S. etc. Result, general depression and nothing done'. Actually something was done because it was as a result of this meeting that Lady Sybil requested Dr Fleming's resignation.

Lady Muriel finally arrived in Petrograd on 25th April, after what seems to have been a more or less Royal Progress through Norway, Sweden and Finland. The winter had not been kind to her. She had been generally unwell and had been working hard, both on the Committee in London and at her own kitchens. Her friend thought that 'she looked fairly fit but seemed thinner and had aged. But it is wonderful to have somebody to talk things over with and who comes with a fresh unprejudiced mind; chock full of ideas, more inclined to act, and act on impulse, than to discuss'. One may take note of Lady Sybil's point of view and we also have the testimony of the English Diarist (whom we will meet again): 'I have made great friends with Lady Muriel Paget. I find her charming and also efficient. The Anglo-Russian Hospital was in splendid isolation and she has already made it more human and more useful'.

The next hurdle to be overcome was the organisation of the field hospital, which seems to have been much delayed by the customary red tape. Here Lady Muriel was magnificent. She cajoled everyone into submission by never taking No for an answer and that certainly applied to her medical staff. *Her* hospital must be attached to the Guards, that élite army who were instantly recognisable by their white belts. Subsequently she had occasion to regret this decision and the unit was transferred back to the 8th Army, but that is another story. However, having a mandate to 'go to the top' she got things done and within the month the second great event in the history of the A-R H. took place.

The Tsarina herself visited the hospital and on this occasion she brought all four of her daughters. The photograph which is reproduced on the opposite page must surely be amongst the proudest memorabilia of the hospital, since it includes almost everyone who helped to put it on the map. Mr Jefferson, who brought it home with him, regarded the day's events with somewhat clinical detachment.

'These functions are an awful bore', he wrote; and a few days later: 'visited by another Grand Duchess who is a great friend of mine but what her name is I never can remember'. These were the natural reactions of someone who wished to get on with the treatment of the casualties who simply did not seem to appear at the doors of the hospital. And the reason was self-evident. 'They say there are 25,000 empty beds in Petrograd, so we are hardly needed here. The Womens Suffrage are sending out four lady doctors but they are going to Galicia. They show more sense than our people . . . We ought to be nearer the front'.

Jefferson's impatience would shortly be rewarded. In the meantime one other offical function had to be observed, the Blessing of the Field Hospital, which took place in the courtyard of the Corps des Pages, a sort of amalgam of Sandhurst and the Wellington Barracks in London. Once again the Grand Duchess Vladimir presided at the inspection and there are several photographs to commemorate the occasion. One shows the Bishops performing the blessing standing behind a portable altar with the choir to their left and Sir George and the Dowager Empress to their right. Another, ten of the *dvukolkas* or covered two-wheeled ambulance carts harnessed to some of the 80 horses which had been purchased by the hospital. A third, four of the six motor ambulances which had arrived, by a stroke of good fortune, that very day from Sweden and which 'were minutely inspected by Her Imperial Highness'. Trucks, horses, ambulances, doctors and *sanitars* were all liberally sprayed with holy water and the Icon blessed. They were at last ready to go. The whole consisted of two units, the Mobile Field Hospital or *lazaret* of about 100 to 120 beds and the Casualty Clearing Station or *peredovoy otryad* which was supported by the ambulance carts.

This time there was no delay and four days after they had been blessed my father wrote to my mother: 'We are off at last'.

In Action

The train which puffed out of a sooty goods-yard on the southern outskirts of Petrograd on Trinity Sunday, the 10th June (28th May OS) was 542 yards long according to WDH, who paced it out. The engine was not pulling a Hospital train although its 53 assorted cars, trucks and waggons did contain an entire hospital. On board were Lady Sybil with her medical, nursing and administrative staff, numbering 19 in all, together with 125 *sanitars,* 44 ambulance carts, 105 horses plus their attendant grooms and two mobile field-kitchens. The medicos were WDH, Gould May, Gardner and Mr Harrison the dispenser. Miss Irvine Robertson took 11 sisters and nurses with her. The Russian Red Cross officials were Boris Ignatiev, Baron Meyendorf and a Mr Martens, and of these I will have more to say.

Before leaving WDH took leave of his batman who must have supposed that he was going to his death because, to his embarrassment, 'Simeon kissed my hand: then went on his hands and knees and kissed the floor'. The train proceeded at pedestrian pace: indeed at times the staff got off to stretch their legs and walk alongside it. It took more than 48 hours for them to reach Polotsk, 'a marshy place, very smelly; many mosquitoes (wrote WDH in his diary). Stayed there 3 days and 2 nights in a siding'. Thence they were directed to Voropayevo, midway between Minsk and Pinsk in the Pripet Marshes and about 600 versts from Petrograd.[1]

A word or two about communications may not come amiss at this point. In Russia the railways were All. There were virtually no roads and those that there were became mud-tracks with the spring thaw and appallingly rutted when they eventually dried out. In the forest areas of the Front no roads existed at all and 'corduroy' roads were constructed from felled pine and birch trunks laid crosswise across the track. This term became explicit for both the appearance and the bumpety nature of these roads, which motor ambulances could negotiate but which horse-drawn carts found more difficult.

---

[1] One *Versta* equalled 0.66 of a mile or 1.06 kilometres. So it took them more than five days to cover 395 miles.

By contrast, the German lines of communication were infinitely superior. From Berlin no less than eight double-tracked railway lines fanned out towards the Eastern Front whereas the Russian network was primitive and for the most part, single-tracked. It is therefore not surprising that with all the other supplies destined for the Front, the A-R H. train bearing its field hospital should have taken so long to reach its destination. And having delivered its load of personnel, tents and supplies, carts and horses, it went once more on its humble way.

Hospital trains were in a different class. There were said to be 300 of them in operation at the Front, each consisting of 29 carriages. Equipped for lying and sitting casualties and with facilities for emergency operations, they were staffed by the Red Cross. Several had sponsors and Train Number One was the gift of the Grand Duchess Vladimir who had instituted an Ambulance train in the Russo-Japanese War. The next five belonged to the Tsarina and the four princesses. By Royal decree they had priority of passage. Scotland Liddell had served as a medical orderly in such a train during the retreat through Poland in 1915 and in his book *On The Russian Front* he gave a vivid account of how his train was the last to leave a beleagured town before its occupation by the advancing German forces: or rather, the last but one, for always on its heels followed the 'blowing-up' train whose sappers wrecked the lines and bridges and installations as they retreated into Russia proper. In addition to the usual facilities Liddell's own train even had a waggon converted to a sort of village-shop cum post-office where supplies could be bought and Red Cross Sisters would write letters to the relatives of wounded soldiers. The Red Cross General-Commandant had his personal truck (immediately behind the engine) laid out as a cosy bed-sitting room with carpet, hip bath and upright piano.

Nobody pretended that Voropayevo was a very attractive village and the climate was anything but clement. Blunt, quoting Lady Sybil, writes that the party arrived at midnight in pouring rain and bitter cold and were conducted to a long, low bleak wooden hut in which they hung blankets to keep out the icy wind. WDH drew a little sketch of this hut in his diary, showing that it was triangular in section with a door at one end and dormer windows along its sides and he records that it was 150 feet long. 'Good ventilation [he wrote, not apparently in jest] and water from well close by.' There they awaited the ambulance carts which arrived by road the following day, having taken from 6 a.m. to 9 p.m. to cover the 50 versts from the railhead.

The weather was atrocious. 'Next morning (wrote Lady Sybil) we wandered about in mud and filth in search of a place to put our tents, and discovered a sandy spot which would be quite nice *when dry!'* Orders came to move nearer the Front, which was some 15 miles away, but these were then countermanded. Lady Sybil and Ignatiev drove in a carriage through seas of mud, which came up to the horses' knees, to interview the General of the Corps, a six mile journey which took the best part of a day. She was told that before long the Guards would move out of the Reserve Line and would advance to Molodechno where the heaviest fighting was taking place. Until then they should wait at Voropayevo.

Suddenly it was summer. The thermometer rose by 40 degrees, the sun shone, the land dried out — and the mosquitoes and flies burgeoned. So they lazed about and after a few days became crotchety and bored. Lady Sybil on one of her excursions came across a village with a huge steam bath and decided to experience the delights of a sauna. 'We were each given a towel the size of a pocket handkerchief and while I was being well steamed a very fat woman carrying a sponge came up to me. She was the Matron of a field hospital nearby and while I was completely naked she made a low bow and passed into a long sentence of flowery Russian welcoming me to the Front. I, while trying to hide myself behind my handkerchief, tried to think of the right exchange of civilities.' WDH took a depressing view of the situation:

> *June 14.* For several days we have had gorgeous summer weather. We have nothing whatever to do. So far there has been no gun fire and we haven't even seen an aeroplane. The devils seem disposed to leave us here. We are moving heaven and earth to get something better and I hope that in a day or two someone will find a spot where there is some fighting.

WDH's prayer may have been answered, for shortly they were moved to Volki (or Volkolati) over roads which had once more become a morass, for the rain had returned, and which exhausted the horses. Finally to Dorlzumolv, near Molodechno and it was here that disaster overtook Lady Sybil. Let WDH's diary set the stage:

> *June 18.* Town full of Polish Jews: about half of them [i.e. the buidings] brick and all of these absolutely in ruins, apparently from fire or dynamite. Russians say that the town was shelled by Germans and Russians at the same time last September. Looks

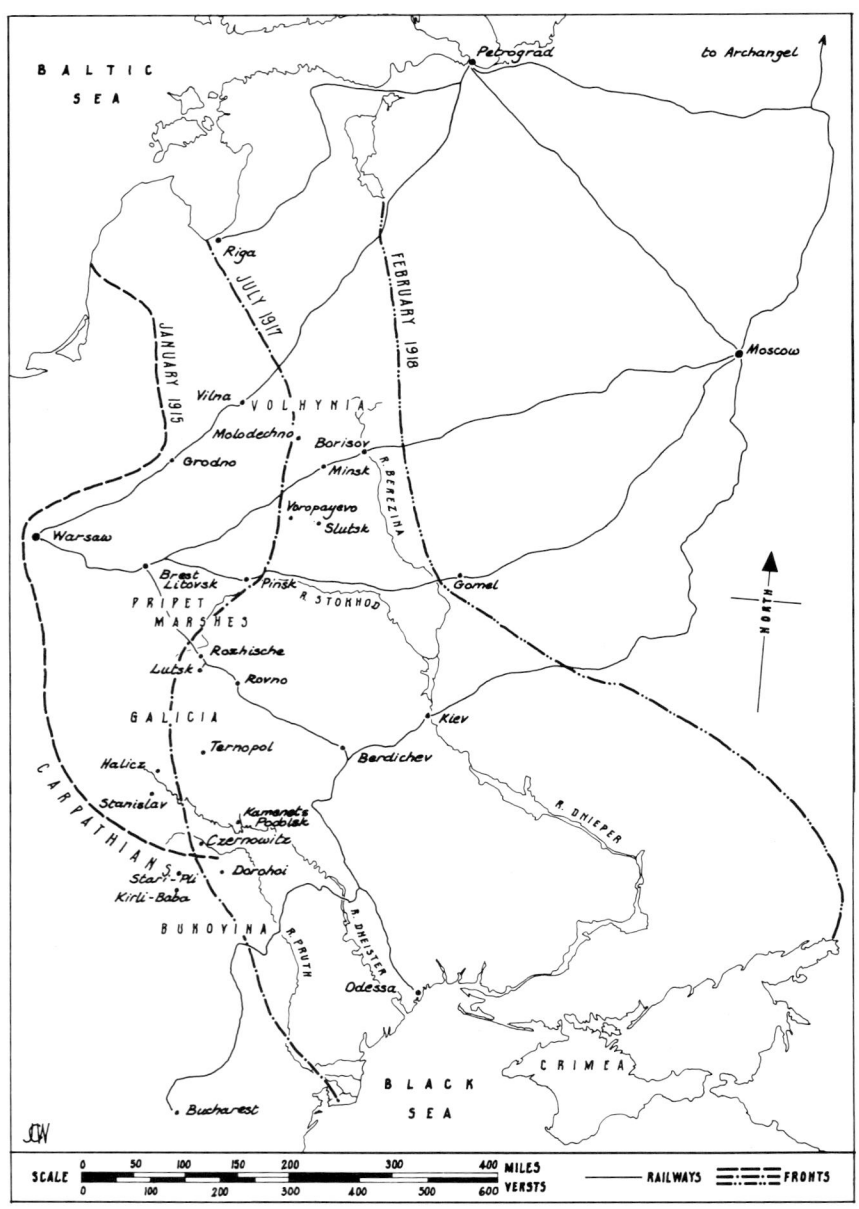

THE EASTERN FRONT

(to us) much more like wilful destruction. Living in a good stone house (formerly a synagogue!) and took meals with the officers. Food excellent.

So, being entirely without the work they had come to do and no doubt after an excellent dinner:

At 8 p.m. walked to trenches to see practise with trench mortars and hand grenades. Party consisted of Lady Sybil Grey, Matron, sisters and 5 or 6 Russian officers. Stood in Bombproof shelter 50 yds behind trenches and watched through narrow slits 3-4" while bomb throwers were used. Many of the officers stood outside but turned their heads when a certain cracking noise was heard. About 9 p.m. hand grenades began. After 4 or 5 series all along trenches, Lady Sybil who was standing on right side of shelter was hit by fragment. Entrance above angle of mouth (left), large enough to admit tip of first finger. Spurting of blood controlled by direct pressure. Hastily driven in carriage to a hut dressing station nearby. Laid on wooden trestle and dressed (wound plugged). Not much shock. Later continued sickness, 6 times during night. Otherwise in good condition. Russian officers very disturbed because I would not operate and remove fragment.

June 19. Condition v. good. Wound looks healthy. Track runs directly backwards and slightly upwards for at least 2½ inches. Bullet *(sic)* not felt. *At 7 p.m.* drove in closed car sent by General to Zymzolabe and found very comfortable [Railway] Car belonging to head of R.X. Train started at once and reached Minsk at 8 a.m. on *June 20.* Here we changed to a 1st class Car given by Gen. Ewart and left at *1 p.m.* Patient getting on well. Some pain (neuralgia) in L. eye. Wound looks well.

June 21. Arrived Petrograd at noon. No one to meet train as they did not expect us till seven. Pt. seems very fit. After lunch X-rayed. Bullet fairly large, deep in skull just below sphenoid and apex of orbit. W. [Waterhouse] very fussed about floor of orbit and difficulty of removal. Cross because he was not asked to take charge.

June 22. 10 a.m. Given C.E. [Chloroform and Ether] by Thompson. Wound plugged with Cocaine and Adren. Bullet easily felt and removed in few minutes without bleeding. Tube drainage. Made a very good recovery and seemed quite herself.

But now let the patient speak for herself, writing in the train on the way to Petrograd, and to her parents:

My Beloveds,

I do hope you won't worry very much when you get a cable to say I was wounded in the face the day before yesterday. Of course it was a piece of most extraordinarily bad luck . . . but it didn't do real damage. An inch to the right it would have shattered my jaw: an inch and a half higher it would have got my eye and might probably have gone into my brain and killed me.

To-morrow they will X-ray me and Mr. Harmer will operate before returning to the front: He is such a dear and *so* kind and very clever, curiously enough one of his specialities is operating on the face, so it is very lucky it is him: but besides that, of all our surgeons I would rather be operated on by him.

I do hope you won't worry at all, for I am marvellously well, very little pain but an immense amount of swelling. Also I have only one eye and 3 quarters of my mouth peeping out of the bandage. I will send you a photograph of the place where it happened. Don't worry, I am happy and comfortable and feel *so* grateful to be alive for I have had a narrow shave. How I wish I could see you.

Miss Irvine Robertson also wrote to Lady Grey:

. . . It is not dangerous and will leave a very small scar, if any, to the side of the left nostril on the cheek.[2] The shock of the impact was tremendous of course and her poor eye and cheek were enormously swollen within the hour. She is — as one expected — as full of courage and spirit as possible, insisting that she has suffered more discomfort than actual pain.

It was only yesterday that Lady Sybil was talking in the highest spirits of our plans. She was riding *astride* ahead of our caravan with a group of Russian potentates and told me she felt just as if we were all in a comic opera.

WDH's subsequent letters to my mother set the seal on a very lucky incident:

June 21st. My dearest
I am back from the front having travelled up with Lady Sybil

2 Her prognosis was correct though at that time she was perhaps somewhat optimistic. Mr Harry Middleton tells me that his mother bore no permanent scar from her injury.

who has been wounded in the face by a hand grenade . . . X-ray shows the bullet deep in the skull and I hope that it will be possible to remove it. But I am anxious about her as there are many complications which may arise. I shall operate to-morrow.
June 25th.
. . . we were able to localise it just below the sphenoid and the next morning I removed it through the wound. Greak luck! because it might have entailed a big operation.

Finally, a letter from Molodechno, to which he had returned:

July 1st. I hear that Lady Sybil is better and will shortly be well enough to return to England.

And so she did; and remained there for the next three months. In spite of its happy outcome I feel compelled to pass some sort of judgment upon this event. Lady Sybil was certainly a VIP but was it right that the senior surgeon, the Matron and one of the important Russian liaison officers should have abandoned the field hospital, which was expected to be in action at any moment, in order to accompany her back to Petrograd? In the event it did not matter much but I cannot help feeling that it was not good for the hospital. WDH was absent from his post for two weeks and when he returned he was met by the resignations of Gould May and Gardner. This may have been coincidental. I do not know and can find no evidence of such a connexion, but it may have inspired his remark (which I quoted in chapter 5) to the effect that he could not blame them since they were all wasting their time. To end on a happier note however, I can record that Lady Sybil called on my mother in London and, hearing of this WDH wrote: 'Glad that you saw Lady Sybil and found her all right. She is a very nice woman and extremely popular here. She seems to have made a great tale about my services which of course will be useful'.

The rôle of the Russian Red Cross in the work of the Anglo-Russian Hospital deserves a special mention in this account. It was fundamental to everything that was achieved though, like everything else which I have attempted to portray, there were problems. Initially Mr Polutsov was the one who mattered. He was one of the five Head Officials of the RRC and he was given the task of assisting the conversion of the Dmitri Palace into a hospital. Once again it is necessary to emphasise that his appointment was a measure of the political importance of this hospital and he was able to assure Lady Sybil that . . . 'all the authorities are behind us and that we are to take top priority'. All accounts agree that he could not have been more helpful and when, because of his age, he had to give up this job everybody was extremely sad. I do not doubt that he is present in some of my illustrations and he must surely have taken part in the ceremony of the Blessing of the Field Hospital. It is my loss that I can not identify him. His deputy at that time was Colonel Fenouk, whom Lady Sybil described as her 'slave': and no doubt he was; but he too has to remain an impersonal figure.

When the field hospital set off on its journey towards the Front, the RRC liaison officers became of much importance since it was their job not only to provision the hospital but also to arrange with the local Commanders where it should be established to do its work. Three men in particular require description and in a way they were as different in character as the Three Ladies whom I described in chapter 3.

First there was Count Boris Ignatiev. I cannot put an exact age to him though he cannot have been more than 30 or so, and he was certainly much younger than his deputy, a fact which gave rise to some incrimination. Lady Sybil liked him but Lady Muriel described him as 'a most obstinate, pig-headed cockshure young man and not quite a gentleman'. (She also accused him of 'treachery' on one occasion). Baron Meyendorf's opinion was that he was 'a man-about-town, but the wrong end of the town!', and there may be some confirmation of this view in an entry in WDH's diary:

> The burning question is whether the Russian Red X are trying to get rid of Ignatieff. There is much gossip and hints about his morals but none of them have any evidence and probably the whole thing is organised by the German influence —? with Meyendorf and Martens in the lead.

This entry brings out quite clearly the schism, which we have noted before amongst the aristocracy in Petrograd, between the pro-Allied Russians and the pro-German Russians. Leaving that aside however, I must record a further entry in the diary when, after a flaming row in which everyone offered their resignations to poor Lady Sybil, WDH wrote: 'Ignatieff apologised for his conduct, *hithero unkown!*' Maybe he was, as they said in those times, a bit of a cad; but WDH wrote

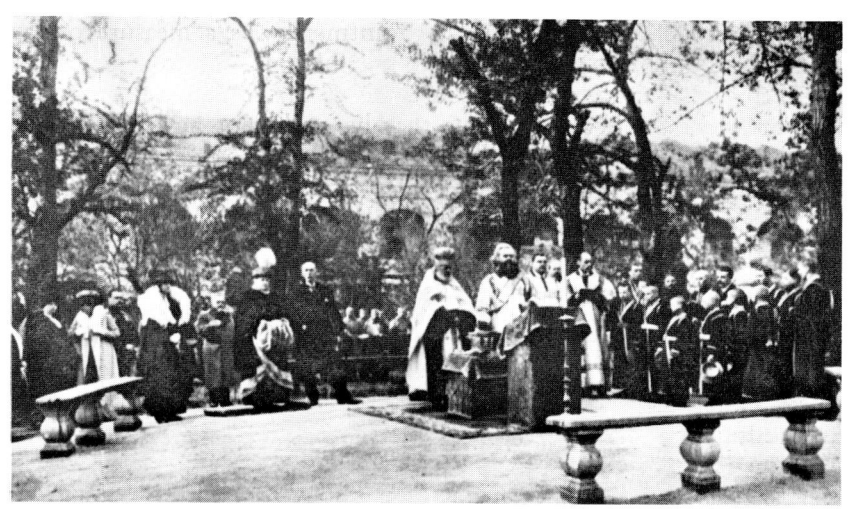

THE BLESSING OF THE FIELD HOSPITAL

generously of his abilities when the fighting began. Moreover one must grant him a considerable degree of spirit.

On 11th August 1916 he sent his Report on the situation at Rozhishche to Lady Muriel (who was then in Petrograd) and asking for instructions. He wrote with some affection, ending his letter: 'I apologise I don't write myself but am afraid you wouldn't read my handwriting, so dictate the letter to my friend Blavdzievich'. Exactly one month later, having received no reply and in obvious pique, he took his pen in hand and tried again, this time in a language with which he was more familiar:

> *Chère Lady Muriel. Ce n'est pas gentil que vous n'avez pas répondre à mon dèpache. J'avais des affaires de famille très importantes à Petrograd que j'ai ajournées pour avoir le très grand plaisir de vous voir à Kieff. Mais, ne recevant aucune rèponse de vous, j'ai dècidé de partir directement . . .*

Reading such letters 65 years later, it is easy to smile: to attempt judgment is another matter. But when Lady Muriel asked the Foreign Office the following year for recognition of the services of her Russian advisers, she added 'and the *smallest pin* for Ignatieff'.

Baron Meyendorf was Ignatiev's deputy. Whether he was really pro-German seems to me doubtful but there is no question about his ancestry and of some suspicion with which he was regarded. Lady Muriel was her customary blunt self: 'Why on earth is M. here at all, working under Ignatieff?'. 'After lunch (wrote WDH) Lady M. persuaded Gen. Bezstrazof to send Ignatief home in 24 hours.' Thereupon the Baron handed her his resignation. Fortunately there was an air-raid during the argument and the matter was forgotten. But Lady Sybil had to hold the fort. She liked Meyendorf too [she liked everybody!] but as usual she recognised his failings, observing that he was 'a brilliant orator, a philosopher, cynical and amusing in a quiet way: a man of letters, not of the sword'. Martens is a more shadowy figure, whose name crops up here and there and who does not seem to have to have been on very good terms with Ignatiev. Apart from the fact that he was 'a diplomat with a nervous twitch of the eyes' he has left little imprint upon the records.

The third of the RRC officials whom I have to mention was, from a biographer's point of view, the most interesting. A wealthy young man of 24 who had recently spent two years at Cambridge, he joined the field hospital chiefly as an interpreter though as things turned out he found himself deeply involved in the Battle of Kirli-Baba with the young Dr Thompson — an experience which may have proved too much for him. By name Alexis Homiakov, he was said to be a typically cosmopolitan Russian intellectual whose interests were art, philosophy and religion. 'He has inexpressibly sad and dreamy eyes, is utterly bored with life and would like to become a monk were it not that he is shortly to be married. And this too bores him inexpressibly'. Lady Sybil's description of him did not prevent Jefferson writing that 'he has had much strife with Flavelle by all accounts' and even WDH could hardly abide his indolence. 'He looks at you with those eyes of his, eyes whose lids come half over them as if it were too much trouble to keep them open and which seem to say: Don't worry — when *you* understand life as I do, you will realise that today, tomorrow or a 100 years hence is all the same.'

I have to confess to a sneaking liking for this young man. It cannot have been all that easy to produce supplies for an unknown number of casualties in a centre of changing fortunes and for a unit which was operating on a quasi-official basis. He was quite evidently out of his depth, for during the Carpathian campaign, Lady Sybil unburdened herself to Lady Muriel:

Homiakoff is leaving for good now. He wrote to tell me he

had got married . . . so perhaps its natural. The little I saw of him in Kieff makes me believe he is useless. He is a very pleasant boy but utterly lazy and frequently says he has done a thing or made an arrangement when he has done absolutely nothing. Matron says that down at the Field he left them without a morsel of food and patients coming in continually. Colonel Count Cheremieff, who was here the other day, says he is known to be absolutely hopeless. He can't help it, because he is a dreamer. . .

No wonder he may have preferred marriage! At any rate he now more or less bows out of my story.

Lady Muriel had arrived in Petrograd towards the end of April 1916 and therefore missed the official opening of the hospital, which had taken place on 1st February; but, as already described, she had played a considerable part in getting the field hospital off the ground and she was present at its Blessing. Having seen it on its way for Voropayevo and Molodechno she took off herself with Fleming to Kiev. Doubtless she had advance knowledge of General Brusilov's great offensive which opened in the region of Lutsk on 4th June, about 250 miles to the south and in which area she thought that her hospital could be of service. It was there that she had her first sight of real war, having previously only seen the wounded tended in her own well-equipped wards in Petrograd. 'Here the casualties lay in their hundreds, in the public squares, not bandaged nor drugged but still in the agony of their fresh wounds. The dying lay there beside the dead, their faces black with flies . . . The day was hot, the stench almost unendurable.' I quote but a fragment of her own account of this, her Baptism of Fire, not to minimise a situation which was all too familiar to those who had been in the line for almost two years but to explain the effect it had upon her: which was that a properly equipped hospital unit should be positioned where it could do a proper job.

So she determined that the field hospital in the north should come south where it might do better work. But war is unpredictable and the arrival of a considerable number of wounded at Molodechno, the lack of transport for such a move and the unexpected injury to Lady Sybil, made the transfer impossible at that time. The defection of Gould May and Gardner, just before things hotted-up, left WDH on his own 'except for a dentist and a dresser', a fact which distressed him intensely. Fleming came up to help him and it is on record that they were at work for four nights and days with very little cessation. For a

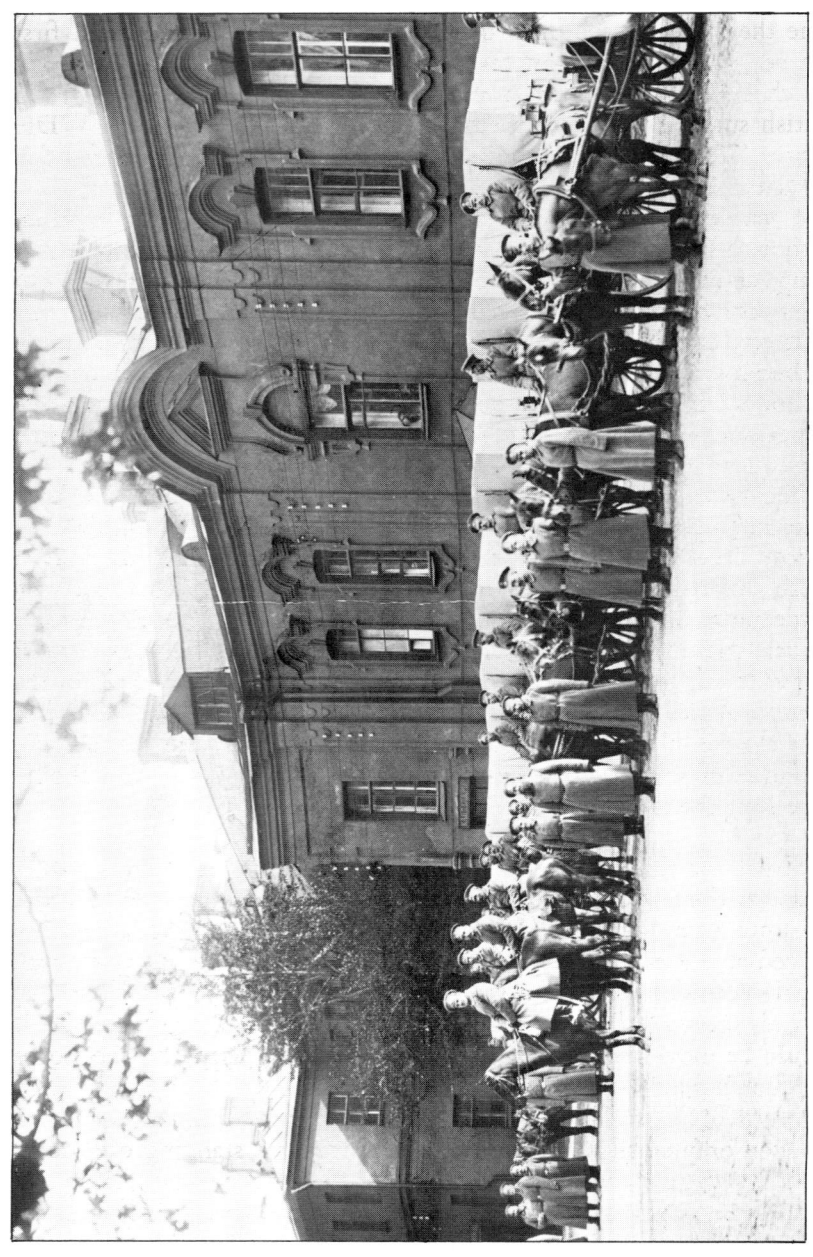

THE PARADE OF THE FIELD HOSPITAL

time they were in the thick of it, as the casualties poured in; at first not so grave but later on (as an article in the *BMJ* made clear and which I quote in a later chapter) the Russians learned to trust the British surgeons and sent them the more seriously wounded. WDH quotes '701 cases, 80 operations, 28 deaths, mortality 4%' for this particular week.

It was about this time that Lady Muriel wrote to my mother. Although this letter has not survived it must have said some very nice things about WDH because he later commented: 'I thought that your letter sent by Lady M. was the loveliest token you had ever sent me. I felt very conceited when I read it'. He certainly needed some cheering up because his ear was 'behaving very badly, much discharge and for 48 hours I had intense pain and quite thought I was in for a mastoid operation'. It recovered, though he was not spared the operation on a subsequent occasion.

The astonishing fortitude of the Russian peasant-soldier has been remarked upon before in this narrative. 'Their bravery is unthinkable (wrote Pares); when there is any reference to the future they say it doesn't matter.' *Neechevo* — a wonderful word, conveying a spectrum of meanings on the same theme: It doesn't matter, It's nothing, Don't bother, Never mind, Not to worry. By extension perhaps, *c'est la guerre!* It implied too a sort of fatalistic hopelessness, and even, in the context of the 1940's, 'Don't you know there's a war on?' Such had been the toll of 1915 that when WDH commented upon the splendid physique of some of the Russian Guards, he was told: 'You should have seen the men we had. They are all gone now . . .'.

About the time WDH returned to Molodechno after Lady Sybil's accident, the air-raids began. This was a new experience and gave rise to some heart-searchings. With German efficiency the aeroplanes arrived at 4 a.m. and 6 p.m. precisely, bombing the railway station. WDH considered it wrong that the hospital, covered with large red crosses, should be located so close to the station and suggested that it should be moved some way distant. This did not appeal to the Corps Commander who saw the obvious advantage of sheltering under its umbrella. Nobody bothered too much about the aeroplanes: they dropped only small bombs and everyone enjoyed standing outside to see the dog-fights which developed between the German planes and the few Russians which went up to intercept them. Zeppelins however were another matter. There was a real fear, almost an hysteria, when the cry 'Zeppelin' was heard. 'Those who didn't fear shrapnell or bullets were terrified of the things which tumble from the sky.'

As the air-raids increased, they moved the hospital into a convenient wood about a mile away and here they were inspected by General Bezobrasov and Colonel Glinka of the Guards Regiment and by a Professor Willheminov (or possibly Veliaminov) who was the senior Red Cross official on this section of the Front. He had many hospitals under his care, apart from the A-R H. and one of these was actually being run by Colonel Glinka's wife. Described by Lady Muriel as 'an old cross-eyed man with long side-whiskers' we can identify him in WDH's diary as 'Old Whiskers'. Cross-eyed or not, the Professor had an iron will and when, a few weeks later at Rovno, the hospital found itself once again in the middle of a large camp which was being bombed incessantly from the air, Lady Muriel and her doctors (together with Mrs Glinka) demanded that 'Old Whiskers' should allow them to move to safer pastures. His reply was to accuse the British of cowardice and, as one might suppose, this was enough to make them stay where they were. 'Suggestion not well received (I read in WDH's diary) so decided to stay..' They got round the problem in a manner which WDH claims was their own invention. They raised earth-walls about three feet high around their largest tents (the casualty wards, the operating theatre, the sleeping quarters for the staff) so that they were protected from the effects of blast, though not of course from a direct hit. A small packet of snapshots, which I found amongst WDH's papers, clearly show some of these protective walls. In addition they sloshed mud and branches of trees over their tents. Nevertheless some 80 persons were killed in the camp on one day and although the nurses' sleeping tent was riddled with shrapnell none were injured.

On 5th July they arrived at Rovno where WDH unexpectedly found Fleming walking in the street. They motored together to Lutsk, 'a fairly large and dirty town with many houses all along the *chausée* in ruins and a large Castle also in ruins'. Then to Rozhishche where the second field hospital was at work under Flavelle and Jefferson and where they found the village absolutely destroyed in the recent fighting and the station being bombed daily. The place being untenable they moved back to Lutsk and there the quantity of troops, guns, ammunition and equipment passing through the town staggered WDH. 'Everything points to a big attack in a day or two' he recorded: and before very long this became all too apparent.

The Battle of the River Stokhod was one of those sharp short engagements, unknown on the Western Front and scarcely mentioned in the official histories, but which nevertheless is of importance in any account of the activities of the Anglo-Russian Hospital. To the south of the Pripet Marshes there is a sort of watershed; some streams running northwards towards the Baltic, others southwards towards the basin of the Danube. The Stokhod ran north. Here, both the Russian and the German armies thought that they might be able to break through to better country beyond. In the event neither succeeded. The battle lasted only four days (28th to 30th July) but Colonel Count Cheremetev recorded that 'the Field Hospital co-operated with remarkable bravery in saving the lives of many wounded under heavy bombardment'. Lady Muriel herself, 'for the valour, self-abnegation and humanity shown by her under heavy fire' was awarded the Medal of St George (2nd Class). It is a pity that for these crucial few days WDH's diary remains a blank, except to record 538 wounded, 74 operations, 21 deaths. No doubt he was too busily engaged to write it up.

When the field hospital left for the Front, Waterhouse remained in Petrograd with Jefferson and Marshall each in charge of one of the two surgical wards in the Palace. It soon became apparent to Lady Muriel that the hospital could be better deployed in the battle zone. How the second field hospital was organised and what it achieved is best told in Jefferson's own words.

> *June 15th* [Petrograd]. There has been terrible fighting on the Southern Front. Lady Muriel Paget and Fleming went down there to see things for themselves. They are so terribly in need of doctors that Fleming has remained behind and Lady Muriel returned to organise an emergency hospital to leave on Saturday. Flavelle has gone down already to be with the motor column. I am to go down with four sisters and Lady M . . . We shall be under canvas and will help with the 200,000 wounded struggling there.

> *June 16th.* Had a very busy day getting things for the hospital. I got all our outfit and six tents at the HQ Store of the Russian Red Cross, an admirable place. They will be delivered here to-morrow evening.

Being young and enthusiastic he could not resist taking a dig at the first field hospital, which had left three weeks before, drawing a neat comparison between the speed with which he had collected his material and the length of time it had taken to get the other off the ground. 'They are off to-morrow — at long last!' he had written to his wife on 25th May. 'Ages getting ready and the joke of the Mess. Exactly where they are going is not known but it is about 50 miles behind the Front, well out of range of everything, including patients I should think!' This opinion proved correct, as we have seen, and led to Lady Muriel's visit to Kiev and her determination 'to get closer to the enemy' — one of Mr Churchill's favourite expressions in both World Wars.

Jefferson's unit consisted of himself and four sisters but he had three motor ambulances and their drivers to look after as well. The country around Kiev impressed him greatly after the barrenness of the north and the people too he found much more charming than those in Petrograd. 'We have attracted a good deal of attention here, being taken for French or Belgians but never English. I spend a lot of time emphasising that we are English.' He wasn't much impressed with the living conditions however. 'We thought when we left Petrograd that we were going to the country and would have all sorts of good things to eat. We have had a rude awakening.'

An even ruder one was to follow and again I cannot do better than record his own account of the events which soon took place. After a spell under canvas, the casualties became too heavy and the unit was moved into a barracks outside Lutsk. A photograph shows a grim square brick building three stories high and we are told that it was intended for the reception of 200 patients. Before long this was increased to 700 and for a few days there were no less than 1400 wounded in this building.

The extra cases were stored under the roof and in the cellars, lying in every conceivable attitude and seen at night it was like The Inferno. The groans of the patients, the shadows thrown by the swinging lanterns, the whitewashed walls, the straw on the floor, on which the unfortunate fellows lay with their blood-splashed bandages; and the heavy atmosphere, heavy with the smell of blood, dirty wounds and bodies, was most extra-ordinary. The wounded came in by rail — on a narrow gauge and in trucks drawn by horses; and here they all lay dead and dying mixed together. It was terrible; but it was an experience I wouldn't have missed for anything. In the past seven days I've dressed 340 major wounds and done thirty-three operations. Our 8th Army must have lost 15000 men, the Guards the same: only *our* army has succeeded while the Guards have failed. The wounded lying about almost in heaps have been astounding.

The Big Push faltered, was held and stagnated. In the lull that followed, Jefferson visited WDH at Rozhishche and after seeing the first field hospital, had this to say to his wife: 'They have been very busy too, but with all their huge equipment they haven't done as much as our little band so we are very proud'. Justifiably; and he richly deserved the decoration which he later received for his work at the Stokhod.

Soon, the first field hospital moved southwards and Lady Muriel came up to Rozhishche to organise the change. They all travelled on a Staff Train — 'very luxurious' — to Minsk and onwards by night: but during the night the train was reversed because it would have passed within ten versts of the front line. There was a wide détour through Borisov on the Beresina River and here at dawn WDH was able to reflect upon the historic site where Napoleon had paused in the terrible winter of 1812 and during the retreat from Moscow. The next day they arrived at Berdechev, 'the capital of the Jews where there is a large undergound town in which are hidden most of the stolen articles in Russia'. I quote this from the diary though I have to admit that it sounds very much like a piece of the anti-Semitism which was current at the time.

That there were grounds for such an accusation however is borne out by a complaint made in December 1918 by Mr Picton Bagge, the British Consul-General in Odessa. By then of course the Armistice had been signed but the Allies were still sending forces into Russia in order to try and contain the Revolution. In the Ukraine there was utter chaos and the price of everything, particularly food, had rocketed. 'Every Jew is doing a roaring speculation (wrote Bagge): 90% of them are very anti-Ally & carrying on a violent propaganda. I hear this on all sides. They are most dangerous & insidious. They have made millions out of Russia's disorders & sufferings.' Whatever may have been the case in the Ukraine in 1918 it was certainly different in Galicia in 1915. In his novel *The Dark Forest,* Hugh Walpole (who was writing from his own personal experience), describes the situation as he found it in a Jewish village afflicted by cholera when he went there with a mobile soup kitchen:

> Near the ruined town-hall we found a company of fantastic creatures awaiting us. There were many children but there were

also many old men with long tangled hair, bare bony breasts and slobbering chins. I thought that I had seen nothing more terrible at the war than the eager pitiful docility with which they moved to and fro in obedience to our orders. A dreadful, broken, creeping submission . . .

But let us leave such contentious matters aside and proceed with the narrative.

During the move south WDH made some observations about the country through which they were travelling: 'The crops here are nearly ready to cut. The straw is 6 ft. high in places and the ears are very long, as many as 30 seeds. It is a vast country and very little of it is cultivated'. Shortly afterwards however, there is an account of a little incident which is worth a mention:

Stopped for petrol and took photos of Austrian [prisoners] Camp. Hid camera on seat of car from where it was stolen — ? by police agent. The next day it was returned by order of the Governor, Col. Count Federicks, by an agent (a wild fellow) and his dog. Camera much damaged without lens or finder. Told that small boy of five had stolen it. Next day lens returned.

Two days ago we rode about 10 miles to see a place nearer the front [for a possible site for the field hospital]. Rather a dismal spot in a large marshy place, 10-12 versts behind the firing line. A Russian village is not unlike what one sees in Switzerland, i.e. a collection of low wooden houses, mostly with turf roofs and nearby the usual tumbledown cowsheds, but everything is much more untidy and poor than with the Swiss. As a rule there is no church and the main street is only a track between the houses. The people look poorer even than their houses: poor clothes, poor health, dirty, with miserable children. But I expect we are in a very poor part of Russia so that one ought not to generalize too much.

The reference to Austrian prisoners is of interest, if only because they were treated by the Russians in an entirely different manner from their German counterparts. Both WDH and Jefferson remarked upon this in their letters, the latter saying that the Austrians seemed to have little stomach for the fight and that they were only too pleased to be given agricultural and supply jobs by their captors. By contrast many of the German officers shot themselves, rather than be taken prisoner and, as for the rest, 'they go to Siberia, a splendid place for the whole German nation!'

Waterhouse came down from Petrograd to replace WDH at Rozhishche. He left with reluctance. 'I have found the time very interesting (he wrote) and everyone, even Meyendorf in his speech said, "Pity he is going".' Then he added (not for the first time I am sorry to record) in a gloomy mood: 'the man that Ignatieff has found to replace him is a nonentity. The hospital will have to be closed soon I think'. There were sound reasons for his fears. Waterhouse reported that Jefferson, at Lutsk, had gone on most well-deserved leave to see his wife (who was before long to give birth to a son) and had been replaced by Dr Rosher, the pathologist. The Russian Red Cross were annoyed — not unreasonably one must admit — 'because we have only one doctor there in the hospital and no more are coming out from England'. Furthermore when WDH arrived in Petrograd he found that 'Aspland has been playing tricks, which is a pity as we had settled to ask him to be CO'. This enigmatic remark finds confirmation too in one of Jefferson's letters, in which he wrote: 'There seems to be more trouble with Aspland but what it is all about it is difficult to know. He seems to be . . . very bad-tempered and egotistical.'

Suddenly and on impulse apparently, Lady Muriel decided to leave for the front. The date was 22nd August, but then we read:

> *Aug 24.* Lady M. back again — unexpectedly! Talked all day about what to do. She wants to move Field Hospital to Kief but Guards want to take it over. Ignatief never goes near it and is playing a deep game, goodness knows what! Decided to go slow: get rid of Ignatief. Send Fleming home. That I must stay till someone else is found. Curse it!!

And that was the very last entry made by WDH in his diary.

Lady Muriel went to Kiev: Fleming went to England; Ignatiev disappeared; Flavelle, returning from leave, took over as Commandant. The centre of action descended on the Bukovina, where the Carpathian mountains made the natural frontier between Russia, Hungary and Roumania. As the autumn weeks closed in towards winter on the Pripet Marshes, the fighting shifted southwards and it was agreed to base the field hospital in the neighbourhood of Czernowitz (now Chernovtsy) and to establish a mobile motor column near Stari-Pli for the evacuation of casualties, nearer the Front. Lady Muriel took the decision to put this in the charge of Mr Peter Keeble, whose name features in Appendix 3 as one of the chauffeurs attached to the hospital. Bernard Pares was in the same area at this time and gives an account of the brisk engagements which took place and of the difficulties of moving the ambulances over the 'corduroy' roads which had been constructed. Both he and Hugh Walpole, who was also there, helped — some say hindered! — the operations of this unit. The local Hungarian population had fled and the Slav contingents in the Austro-Hungarian forces were defecting in huge numbers. In one of his letters, WDH writes of a Russian unit which, being surrounded, wished to surrender to the attacking 'Austrians': only to be informed that it was they (being Serbians) who craved surrender. It must have been a real mess.

In November there was another of those short, sharp battles which again has found no place in the official histories. For four days and nights there was heavy fighting and even heavier casualties near a village with a name which might well have come out of *The Arabian Nights* — Kirli-Baba; and it was here that Lady Muriel found Dr Thompson, assisted by the dreamy Homyakov, in one tent 'entirely surrounded by mud and with no stretchers nor anaesthetics', dealing with the wounded. In the four days, we are told, he treated 400 casualties; and was very properly decorated for so doing with the Cross of St George. Commenting on this coveted award in a letter to Lady Muriel, Jefferson added that a Chaplain called Pritchard had got a St George's Medal 'but for what reason is not quite clear'. The only other mention of this Reverend gentleman comes in a letter from Lady Sybil to Lady Muriel, in which she was lamenting some of the failings of the new Commandant. 'Flavelle fairly lets himself go about Pritchard. Says that Bryden [another of the chauffeurs with the motor column] is an honest, decent fellow but is under the influence of the canting Priest, that loathsome Pritchard etc. This is where Flavelle is bad: he has no control over his temper.'

Lady Muriel now went off on her own, seeking a new site for the hospital, demanding interviews with Corps' Commanders and so on. Before he decided to pack up and go home, Dr Gould May had quoted, of this mercurial woman, 'you have to be a bat to know what the bats are flying after'; and even WDH, in a rare moment of exasperation and when he was waiting for her permission to allow him to return to England, wrote to my mother: 'Lady M. has not turned up yet and everyone is very excited about her. If I were her good man I should buy a big stick and see whether that had any effect!' Of course Sir Richard was not that sort and when Lady Sybil returned to Russia in October he entrusted her with a 24-page letter (not knowing that his wife was at that time in imminent danger at the front) describing, with plans, a Zeppelin which had been brought down in north London. This letter also included the unique paragraph:

> On Monday morning John drove me to the station in the donkey-cart. The distance being 1¼ miles and the donkey being 34 years old, we allowed 40 minutes but actually did it in 35; the formula being: $\frac{V}{D} = \delta + 1$, where V = Velocity of flight (in miles per hour), D = distance (in miles) and δ = the donkey's age (in years).[3]

With the hospitals at last properly engaged and working hard, the London Committee made a major fund-raising effort. A matinée was organised and Queen Alexandra herself was present. Not only that, for by chance the Grand Duke Michael, the younger brother of Tsar Nicholas II and in whose favour the Tsar abdicated in March 1917, was in Britain and he too was able to attend. The best talent of the day gave their services: Gertie Miller, Gladys Cooper, Phyllis Dare, Harry Tate, Charles Hawtrey; and 'a band of ladies, including many society beauties, appeared to reap a rich harvest by the sale of programmes'. The Secretary of State for War (Mr Lloyd George) was to have spoken during the interval but his place was taken at the last moment by a deputy 'who made his stage debut like a junior curate saying his piece'. His name was Winston Churchill and I cannot help wondering whether he may have recollected this occasion when he wrote the words which I have quoted at the beginning of chapter 3. The matinée raised £1100.

It was about this time that Lady Muriel, on the moonlit platform of Rovno station, composed her rash telegram to Lord Cheylesmore more or less demanding the immediate despatch of a hundred ambulances (a brief reference to which was made earlier in my account). It was doubly unfortunate because she also sent a copy of her

---

[3] Blunt, *Lady Muriel*. Pamela Lady Glenconner not only remembers the donkey-cart but made a beautiful little sketch of it for me. My regret is that it is not possible to reproduce it here.

telegram to the Press, a more honest move perhaps than the contemporary 'leak', but none the less embarrassing to the Committee who were having some difficulty in raising the money necessary to keep the hospitals in being. Lord Cheylesmore found Lady Muriel not only difficult to keep track of (as so many others did) but a very poor book-keeper as well. We find him writing on 8th September:

> I am afraid you put a wrong construction on my letter. The Committee did not imply any mismanagement; but they were all exercised in their minds as to what was happening, as they had received no reports or statement of accounts and they did not know who was in charge of the Hospital . . . They were certainly frightened when they saw it announced in the papers that the Hospital was appealing for funds to supply 100 motor ambulances with the staff for each, which they never sanctioned and knew they could not supply.
>
> I can assure you there was nothing personal in my letter and the Committee thoroughly appreciate your energy and the work you have done. As we have received no accounts for months, the Committee thought the best thing to do would be to send out someone responsible for them. There was no reflection on you in this, and they never for a moment thought that you would take it so seriously as to threaten to resign . . .

One cannot doubt Lord Cheylesmore's word, but to *resign?* Impossible! A sort of trump-card perhaps, but I prefer to think of Lady Muriel, by then on another tack, shrugging of His Lordship's reply with a 'What's all the fuss about' or even *neechevo!*

It would be foolish to pretend that there were not some in the London Committee who disagreed with the manner in which Lady Muriel ran their affairs. A letter from a friend of hers reveals the fact: 'Roderick Jones and Lady Gladstone, they say, want your head but they at once saw how impregnable your position was when I gave them the facts. The despatch from the F.O. sent to the Committee praised you and your work to the skies. This of course was based on a despatch of mine sent from Kieff and has apparently knocked the ground from under their feet!'

Some sort of assessment of the state of the hospital at the end of its first year now seems to be called for. From the beginning Dr Andrew Fleming had never been popular as a Commandant and when Dr John

Flavelle was appointed in his place (after WDH had done the job for a matter of weeks) he proved to be even less so. The doctors were unquestionably kittle cattle, as Mrs Lindley remarked, but why there should have been such internecine squabbles between them I cannot say. Lady Sybil did a splendid job in organising the establishment of the hospital and a truly magnificent one in keeping it going during the uprising in Petrograd. Had she not been wounded and had she not had to return to England when her father lay dying, things might have gone better. But that is anticipating events. And Lady Muriel: but how can one 'assess' Lady Muriel? If she had gone out at the beginning, if she had not had so many other interests, if she had been a better manager and book-keeper, if she had not been so determined to be in the front line all the time, if she had got on better with her Russian advisers . . . There are too many imponderables.

So let me pause awhile in my chronological account and consider a more personal aspect.

Belles Lettres

Since this Essay is dedicated in part to my Father, it is proper that I should devote a chapter for the most part to him alone.

When I first saw the 54 letters which he had written from Russia I had to arrange them in chronological order and this was not so simple an operation as might be supposed. Father numbered them and so did my mother. Usually they were double-dated with both the Russian OS nomenclature[1] and the English date. But this system did not always obtain and in consequence he sometimes appears to be answering a letter which he had not yet actually received. A classical example of the confusion of a particular date is that of the assassination of Rasputin. For the Russians it was 16th December; for the rest it was 29th December. A similar problem arose concerning the date of the opening of the hospital. The BRCS record says 18th January but Father's diary states 'Feb. 1'. Blunt, in *Lady Muriel,* writes that it should have been on Sunday, 30th January but that it had to be postponed for two days at the request of the Dowager Empress. A newspaper cutting from the *Westminster Gazette* is simply headed 'tuesday'; so I am inclined to agree that the opening did take place on 1st February. Not that it matters of course, but it does illustrate the difficulty of accurate chronology.

It is a pity that the first letter that Father wrote has not survived because I am sure that he gave an interesting account of his journey from Newcastle to Petrograd. That it did not do so is evident from the fact that his earliest letter bears the number 2, in my mother's handwriting, and because its content implies that it followed a previous one. As it is, this letter is superscribed 'Nov. 29' in one corner and 'Dec. 12' in the other, while the envelope bears not only four postmarks — 1st, 4th, 17th and 20th December — but also a magnificent seal, some two inches in diameter, plonked on by the Censor; and which (who knows?) may one day make it a collector's piece.

---

[1] The OS Calendar was suppressed following the Revolution.

The Russian censorship was very strict and this is not surprising, considering that in 1915 there was a powerful pro-German lobby in Petrograd. For this reason the newly arrived doctors asked the British Embassy if their mail might go home in the Diplomatic Bag: 'but (wrote Father in his third letter) they don't want to be bothered with us'. No doubt this accounts for the fact that in three of his early letters whole sentences are expunged in deep purple ink. And serve him right, if many of his letters written from The Front the following year, may be taken as an example; for they included references to where he was, to which Russian units the hospital was attached and so on, details which would have made any W.W.2 security officer's hair stand on end! But by then an agreement with the Embassy had been reached and one reads: 'I hear there is a bag going out to-morrow', or 'I must end now to catch the bag'.

The Bag was a life-line for those on service. Ordinary letters were taking anything from four to twelve weeks and even the Embassy mail was often held up in Sweden or, on occasion, sunk in the North Sea. It is remarkable that there is such a complete collection of Father's letters to my mother in the circumstances. Of hers to him, not one remains and that for a simple reason. 'I hear that it is very hard to get anything through the Customs. No books or anything allowed. All yours will have to be burnt, which is dreadful.' Poor Father; and what a loss to his biographer!

Father's letters may perhaps be divided, like Caesar's Gaul, into three parts. Most of them begin with an account of what was happening to the hospital and how he himself was getting on. Then there are anxieties about how things were at home, with affectionate, if sometimes obligatory, references to the children. Lastly, a more personal coda in which he expressed his most intimate feelings. I would not wish to reveal such confidences; indeed I find it embarrassing to read, after so many years, much the same thoughts and aspirations as I myself wrote to my own wife during the later war. Perhaps such letters should not have been kept. Yet if they had not been preserved there would have been a most significant hiatus in this narrative.

I will deal with the children first. In the autumn of 1915 Richard was eight and a half, Christopher was five and I was three and a bit. Naturally Father's chief concern was with his eldest son who was at Prep. School at the time and whose progress he wished to know about. My mother provided this no doubt, but as her letters have not survived one has to indulge in some assumptions: '. . . I think you must have helped him with his spelling in his letter to me', for example. On another occasion: 'Richard seems rather a handful and I don't know what sort of time you will have when Mike is his age. Perhaps the others will keep him in order'. Perhaps they did, because in a later letter I see: 'I am sure Mike is being as good as ever'. I doubt that and I can say with certainty that he was wrong when he headed a letter: 'July 3rd Mike's 4th birthday', since I was born on 6th July. Christopher was a bit of a worry because he was suffering from strabismus which necessitated an operation upon one of his eyes. But in the tradition of those times, when Father did write to his children (and there are three such letters in the collection) he always ended: 'Love from your affectionate father, W. Douglas Harmer'.

The Zeppelin raids of 1916 on London alarmed him because he had experience of the effects of the bombs which they cast down and which were of an altogether different order of those dropped by aeroplanes. As a result, Christopher and I were taken out of London and for a time were at Sea View in the Isle of Wight; and there in early June of that year I am able to recall my earliest recollection, a few warships returning to Portsmouth after the Battle of Jutland.

There were also financial considerations which had to be taken into account. At the beginning of 1914 Father was well established as an Oto-rhino-laryngologist and his house in Weymouth Street was becoming too small for his growing family and his growing practice. Accordingly he bought the lease of one of those splendid Crown Estate houses in Park Crescent at the northern end of Portland Place and alterations had already begun at the time of the outbreak of the war. Then everything came to a full stop. So we find him writing: 'Have you done anything to try and get rid of Park Crescent?'; and a couple of months later: 'What are we going to do about 9 P.C.? I suppose you haven't found anyone foolish enough to want it!' Later a spirit of optimism prevailed: 'As regards Pk. Crescent, I think you ought to hesitate before taking the plunge'. The plunge was not taken, but in 1917 the authorities said that unless the house was occupied it would be commandeered for war use and so, in the very deepest part of the war, the family moved in and there remained until bombed out in 1942.

The Letters are full of fascinating little details about stocks and shares and possible investments, though there were occasions on which his enthusiasm was misplaced to say the least. 'I see that the rouble is very cheap. I think we should buy; they are bound to appreciate after the war'. [Thank God he didn't]. But more sensibly: 'I don't think you should sell your Shells. I fancy they will go higher after the war. Someone prophesised that they would go to £10 and in any case they have always paid a fair rate of interest'[2] My mother must have been sensible as well, for in another letter we read: 'How you have managed to invest £1000 since I came out I don't know. It sounds as if you've made a mistake in the amount. Anyway it is very satisfactory and I am not costing very much. I still have some of the original £70 I brought out with me'; and he wrote that nine months after he had left home. But he made up for this later on when he went on a shopping-spree.

> I spent most of the afternoon — over two hours — bargaining with a dirty old Jewish woman about a lace dress and a Chinese shawl which I had unearthed in a dreadful little shop in the Jews Market. Eventually she accepted my price and I got them for 120 roubles less than she wanted. I think the shawl is a bargain and Aspland agrees [he should have known, having been a medical missionary in China for many years] because it is beautiful old silk and worked on both sides. But the lace is much more difficult to price . . . all the same, it is a very beautiful thing and I had quite made up my mind to get it for you. I daren't tell you the price until you have seen it but I said to myself that I must come home with a present really extra-special, to show you that I want you to have what I think you deserve for this long wait alone and for sticking to me in spite of it all.

Some of his contemporaries did not enlist and of them Father was critical: 'I have no sympathy with the doctors at home. They ought to remember that in any other profession they would have to go whatever their financial responsibilities. I can quite understand that it is pleasant to stay at home and reap the profits'.

Like all those serving overseas in time of war, the hospital staff were beset by rumours and in particular were concerned about the Western

[2] This remark (letter of 28th June) may well be the origin of something which became almost a family motto: *You Do Not Sell Shell*. It certainly was wise advice. Mr F. R. Bishop of the Shell Company tells me that in 1916 the £1 ordinary shares were quoted at about £5; so that my mother's 500 shares would have been worth £2500. They actually reached £14.10s. in 1920 and since then have been divided on so many occasions that they would now be represented as 20,736 shares of 25p each. At a market value of £4.25 per share my mother's holding would have been worth £88,128 in 1980.

Front where many of their friends and contemporaries were dying. [By contrast, of the 109 personnel of the hospital listed in Appendix 3, only one is named as deceased.] Sweden was vacillating 'but is likely to remain neutral: Roumania is mobilising and will probably come in next spring, but on which side?' [In fact they came in on the side of the Allies and were immediately gobbled-up by Germany.] In the summer of 1916 Verdun and the Somme were the great talking points and there are many references to these great battles. There was also a rumour of a great naval engagement in the North Sea, which of course turned out to be Jutland. 'The Russians (wrote Father) have much respect for our Navy'; but he did not reciprocate the compliment, adding: 'The Russian navy is no good. Their officers are said to damage their own ships so as to be able to get back to port. The same happens if a little wind springs up when they return *because of storm'.* Again: 'The educated Russian is generally impressed by what our fleet has accomplished: filled with admiration over the way we catch submarines, but several are asking whether the English mean to go on as they hear of a peace party in England & if England fails them, Russia is done'. In writing this to her mother, Lady Sybil added: *'Jamais de la vie,* I swear by every oath I can think of'. In another letter to her sister she returned to the same theme: 'As the months pass, the Russians have an increasing sense of betrayal. Doubts begin to be whispered; can the allies be trusted? . . .'

When the cruiser *Hampshire* went down in the Arctic Sea, drowning Lord Kitchener on his way to Russia, everyone was appalled. 'I cannot get over the stupidity of letting everyone know when he was starting & where he was going. In Pet. everybody knew & I suppose they did in England. The general opinion is that we were terribly imprudent.' These too were Lady Sybil's words and Father wrote in the same vein: 'This is dreadful news about Kitchener! As one of the patients in the wards said to me, "why do you talk about these things beforehand? Why didn't they keep the whole thing dark if he was coming?" But it is a hard piece of fortune and I am very sorry for the Navy. Still, he will emerge as the hero of the war perhaps! In any case it ought to stimulate our people'. There was another rumour too, that the Kaiser had had two operations upon his throat.[3] 'Very improbable (remarked Father drily) as he was supposed to have been shot dead in Brussels last week.'

[3] There may well have been some confusion here with his father, Frederick III, who had died of cancer of the larynx, after several operations.

Throughout the war Russia was literally crawling with spies and this was to be expected since all her Provinces, from Finland in the north, along the Baltic States, down through Poland to the Carpathians and on to Bessarabia, were populated by discontented minorities who had been promised freedom by the Germans and Austrians. In particular there were a large number of German-speaking settlements in the Ukraine. Then of course there was the enormous Jewish population; and whatever was to befall these unfortunate people 25 years later at the hands of the Nazis, it is indisputable that they had had a miserable time under the Tsarist regime and therefore looked westward for a better life. So they constituted a security risk; and rightly so, since many acted as informants in the battle zones and even in Petrograd itself. 'Many (wrote Pares in *My Russian Memoirs*) deserted to the enemy both from the ranks and from amongst the officers.' 'It is difficult to blame them', he added in a despatch to the Foreign Office.

German Intelligence was certainly first-class and in any book about this period of the war one will find accounts of spies and spying. Father's letters are no exception. Although we may perhaps discount tales of candles in cottage windows and the telephone call from the village post-office which immediately preceeded an air-raid, it is worth recording the story of a German Colonel who had been surprised with his entire unit. 'Apparently the order had been given to the Russians to attack at 2 p.m., but the officer had misread the signal and attacked at 2 a.m. When he had captured the German Colonel, the latter complained bitterly that he had not carried out his orders and so had taken him by surprise. He knew quite well when the attack ought to have been made. The Russian officer apologised of course.' Another tale reads much the same. 'When we were in the Ukraine a new [Russian] general was sent to take command. The Germans knew he was coming: bombed the hotel where he and his staff were and incidentally where most of the Russian officers congregated, and killed the lot.'

Then there is a mention of the great explosion in Murmansk in the summer of 1916. The British had sent a large ammunition convoy to this Russian port but, it is said, German agents blew up the whole lot with the virtual destruction of the entire town. There were thousands of casualties and few medical services: the Tsar despatched his own train to succour the injured. Unfortunately the carriages were too broad to traverse the first tunnel on the railway and so this relief operation came to grief with many more dead. Father implied that the A-R H. was involved in this rescue operation, but I have been unable to find any evidence of this among the official records of the hospital or in the letters of Lady Muriel and Lady Sybil. It would be nice to suppose that some of the nurses and doctors had gone on this errand of mercy but if anyone had done so, surely it would have been Lady Muriel herself? I fear the story must be discounted, at any rate as far as the A-R H. was concerned.

A few extracts from Father's letters illuminate what was certainly a sombre year.

The winter of 1915-1916. All are agreed that this was one of the most bitter winters in recorded history, not excluding that of 1812: and this fact has been mentioned in descriptions and quotations in earlier chapters. Here is another variation on the same theme:

> All the prisoners that the Russians have been taking round Riga are still clad in Summer clothes & I believe it to be absolutely true that the Germans are stripping all Russian peasants in order to get their clothes & turning them out into the forests to starve & freeze. The Russians think that Germany had made so sure of getting Riga & having their winter quarters there, with getting command of all the railways before this date, that they had not organised getting winter clothing up to their men.

The following summer. There was a saying which I heard when I was in Leningrad myself, that their year usually consisted of nine months winter and three months waiting for summer. This was unquestionably true of 1916. Apart from a few days in June the weather was atrocious, as indeed it was in Flanders also. Even the White Nights, when there is virtually no darkness and the northern sky normally takes on a lovely beige hue, were few in number. It seemed almost to presage the Gotterdämmerung.

> April 24th. The Neva is still full of floating ice.
> June 20th. Weather appalling. Cold as November. Floods of rain. Roads covered in thick lakes of mud up to the top of one's knee-boots. Motors will be quite useless.
> August 3rd. Still raining hard . . .
> September 29th. It is bitterly cold o'nights and we are shutting down the tents and going into buildings.
> October 15th. Torrents of rain for a long time now . . .

The patients are terrified of anaesthetics & consequently refuse operations. As in England one cannot compel a man to have an operation: the percentage of refusals is bigger because they are terrified of going back to the conditions and experiences which they have suffered.

Le Roy to dinner last night. Says the only compensation a soldier gets if he has lost a leg is the permission of the Govt. to became a beggar.

I don't mind saying now [he had just returned to Petrograd from the Front] that the aeroplanes were the very devil. I was talking to Hands when he was hit in the thigh and I was lying on my face another day when a piece of metal came plug into the ground by my side.

For 3 days at a time there was a roar of big guns every second, day & night. When this goes on the ground trembles, even 10-12 versts from the front. What it is like in the trenches goodness only knows. Why any man stays there passes my comprehension.

I hate looking at the papers now because the Casualty Lists are so enormous . . .

In connexion with 'near misses' he was a little less charitable concerning one of his colleagues (whose name I suppress). 'Dr —, in writing to Lady Muriel, said he was sorry his writing was so shaky but a shell had just burst 3 yards from him, which was rather upsetting. Pure invention of course but I gather most of them believed it.'

Shortly afterwards he wrote about himself: 'Everyone was very nice to me when I left the Field and what impressed me most was when the Russian *sanitars* (about 100 of them) solemnly marched up in line, at dinner time, and made a long speech saying they were sorry to lose me, to which I replied shortly'. I wonder in what tongue he replied? If it were in Russian it would explain the shortness, for he never achieved much in that language though I am sure he did his best. It is on record that only Russian was permitted to be spoken over the telephone, German being totally *verboten,* though Lady Sybil managed to obtain a special dispensation to speak French in connexion with the management of the hospital.

It was not all gloom however and some happier memories occur here and there in the letters. In May, Father attended a sitting of the Duma. 'Everyone very excited and as the President was unable to stop the disorder with ringing of his bell, he adjourned the House. Before resuming he announced that the Russians had broken the Austrian line at Czernovitch and had captured 12,000 prisoners. Loud cheering and then the President told everyone to stand up to show their respect for the men who had fallen and everyone stood in silence for several minutes.' On another occasion he was at the Opera and wrote that he slept through most of the first Act. He was, I regret to add, equally unsympathetic towards the Ballet though he loved the music. I have already mentioned how impressed he was by the inborn ability of the Russians' singing, and there is a nice little snippet in one of the letters where he describes how the drivers of the motor column in the Bukovina were doing their best to compete. Said a Russian Colonel to him: 'Your English have the ear but they do not have the voice'. Fair comment perhaps, even though some of those on the roll appear to have Welsh names.

In June, when the field hospital was waiting for work, he went on a fishing expedition with some Russian officers. There were 'any number of big lakes with quantities of coarse fish. We started by trying a Sein net but as it wasn't very successful they then proceeded to sink some dynamite cartridges which stunned the fish'. This must have been a well recognised method for Liddell has much the same description in *On the Russian Front*. 'There was a lot of wind and nothing but small canoes — very unseaworthy! — to go out and pick up the fish. Great excitement when one of the soldiers was swamped. At one time it looked doubtful if he would make the shore.' He did. Finally, there is a charming little story about one of the Russian medical orderlies: 'One of our *sanitars* asked me whether I could give him any instruments. When he goes back to his village beyond the Urals, he intends to set up practice as the local surgeon'.

Father also had some pertinent observations to make about the Orthodox Church:

> The wealth of the churches must be colossal. Each of them is plastered with ikons — mostly silver, but many of gold with precious stones. Then there are countless silver candle-stands and in one Cathedral (the Kazan) some solid railings with [?posts] as thick as ones leg around the whole side of the church, made of solid silver.

Of the magnificent Easter Service, which was briefly noted in chapter 7, he wrote that he found it 'very interesting, rather depressing and perhaps a little morbid. Very mournful music and the ceremony somewhat gruesome to our mind but very impressive and obviously means much to the people'. He was referring then to the wax effigy of Christ which, having been processed around the church and laid to rest at the altar, appeared to vanish on the stroke of midnight. He drew some conclusions:

> It certainly had the effect of making one realise how little heed is paid to religion in our own country. It must give the Church here a great hold on its people and I think I begin to understand why the Catholics (sic) are more under the control of their priests. It is impossible not to be moved in such an atmosphere. There must be many who are frightened by the seriousness of it all and no doubt it is an influence that is good. I am very glad to have seen some real religion at last.

I wonder if he may also have witnessed something the English Diarist described: 'Walking down the Nevski I overtook a religious procession in the midst of the trams and traffic. Who should be out for a walk but the icon of the Kasan Virgin, who lives in the Kasan Cathedral, accompanied by her own metropolitan with his walking-stick. I followed her into her Church and saw her popped into her frame again. She has a huge emerald on her chest, and a diamond crown'.

When my Father wrote these particular letters he was anything but well. He continued: 'Everyone complains that I look so thin, which annoys me intensely'. Indeed none of the staff enjoyed good health and, as it were in justification of his own, he added: 'I saw Prof. Pares for a few minutes and *he* looks miserably thin & seedy. He has a St. George's X and Medal for work at the front and has had a tough time of it'.

Mr Geoffrey Jefferson also wrote a considerable number of letters to his wife while she was in England; and again after she had been out to Russia and returned home with their new-born son. These letters were also kept and Mr Antony Jefferson has been generous enough to place extracts from 26 of them on tape and allowed me to use them in my narrative. Many interesting details, dates and so on have thereby been incorporated which would otherwise have been missing. No biographer can fail to be impressed by the writings of this young man of 29, who so clearly summed up the situation in which he found himself. His style of writing is altogether more evocative than that of WDH in his own letters.

His first impressions of Petrograd were of a rather seedy city. 'Frankly, very disappointing and not to be compared with Edinburgh or even London. The streets badly paved with cobbles. The best palaces very grand but many shabby. A lot of the shops in the back streets display paintings indicating the goods for sale, as the shoppers are largely illiterate.' Later he was to modify this opinion, 'for Petrograd grows on you'. He wrote that it looked as if he would die of boredom and that there was nothing to do except learn French. 'But tennis may save my life: I'm told that they play up to 11 p.m. in the White Nights. Like all the other Englishmen he was astonished at the singing of the unaccompanied choirs in the churches and he recorded also hearing a battalion of soldiers on the march: 'No bands. They sing as they go with a sergeant-baritone in charge, very well indeed and the songs evidently much more serious than Tipperary'. He went to Lord Kitchener's Memorial Service at the English church, which was a most spectacular affair since it was attended by all the Ambassadors and élite of the City. 'The Sermon was the worst I have ever heard and that is saying a good deal! We all hoped that the Russians did not listen to it nor understood it.'

In his letters he also gave his opinion of most of his colleagues. Over some I must draw a veil, though I have to add that because of the exigencies of the war he came across my father very little and left nothing on record concerning him. Of the two Ladies, he was clearly more impressed by Lady Sybil — 'a very, very charming and sensible woman'. 'Lady Muriel (he regretted) has such silly ideas and is always starting some fresh scheme. She talks about sending out five field hospitals and they can't even get one off. This is two months overdue now! Then she wants to buy a hospital train, as if it were possible to buy a train here. They are short of rolling stock already and it isn't likely that we could get one made. As Gould May says: her head is full of flies.'

Towards the end of his time in Russia, during May and June 1917 and when the work at the base hospital was mainly medical, he had the opportunity of making some interesting visits. With Dr Rosher he went to the Institute for Sera Manufacture which was established in one of the old forts on Kronstadt Island. Here there were horses, dogs, monkeys and a wealth of equipment which impressed him greatly. Equally so was that in Professor Pavlov's laboratory, where the original work on conditioned reflexes in dogs was being done. 'The apparatus, machinery etc. for excluding errors is the most remarkable and ingenious that I have ever seen.' More to his own taste was the Neurological Institute of Professor Poussep to which he had an introduction through a Russian surgeon whose papers he had helped to re-write in English. Reference has already been made in an earlier chapter to his removal of a bullet from the brain of a young soldier and now I find a mention of this achievement in a letter dated 27th May 1917:

> Yesterday I read my paper, 'the Cerebellar Bullet', before the Russian Society of Surgeons of Pirogov at the Mariniski Hospital and had a very interesting evening. They were most kind, talked of the Anglo-Russian *entente* and ended by making me a life-member of the Society. Rather nice, isn't it?

Soon he was to go home. 'My substitute has arrived: a young American from Chicago. [He remains anonymous as far as the records are concerned.] It will be so nice to be with you again but I am very sorry to leave Russia now that I am up against the actual leaving. It really has an extraordinary charm . . . Food is scarce: queues from 4 p.m. to dusk. [And as for the hospital] it is like the old times again . . . As a matter of fact they talk — and talk — and talk — and don't do anything.'

It is quite clear that the authorities, both in London and in Petrograd, would have liked Father to become the Commandant when it was known that Fleming would be returning home in August 1916: and it is equally evident from reading his letters that his sense of duty was struggling against his wish not to be cajoled into doing so. 'I don't want to be asked to take charge because it would mean staying out here indefinitely. Besides, I should hesitate to bring you out because I think the kids want you more than I do for their welfare. *My* wants are so largely selfish.' The pressure continued and it seems he may have been having doubts: 'August 26th. I feel I can't desert the ship when I am wanted. Fleming is going home and I must stay until some new C.O. is discovered. He is still to be found. I feel inclined to tell them to go to Hades and clear out'.

Eventually he came to a decision and for the only time lost patience with Lady Muriel:

Sept 24th. Lady M. is careering about in the South and shows no signs of returning at present. It is very tiresome of her especially as I gave an ultimatum that I did not intend to stay later than to-day. However she knows that I can not leave before she returns and has taken a strong line and said nothing. I suppose she will be back next week and will want to go straight back to England and leave me. I am getting a bit fed-up and there is a limit to my patience.

Much has been said about Dr Andrew Fleming in this Essay and although Father described him on one occasion as 'very fussy', I think it is right to record his ultimate judgment of the man who put the hospital on the map. Writing to my mother, who had clearly sent him a rather depressing account of Fleming on his return to England, Father wrote:

I am very sorry to hear about Fleming. He was very run down, as the result of hard work, and was looking much older than when he came to Russia. He has had a rotten time in many ways and has behaved splendidly, never bearing any malice to anyone. A great many people have been anything but loyal to him . . . But I hope people in England will realise that he was always considering their interests, in fact the best friend the hospital had out here. The trouble has been that each person has seen what they thought would be advantageous to themselves. There has been far too much selfishness. I shall be thankful to get out of it all because I hate being in a job which is complicated by eternal quarrelling. The tales I have had to listen to all day and every day have been sickening. And yet in spite of our stupidity the show has been a success in many ways and Fleming is the only man who deserves any credit. Though you had better not say that I told you so because it is no use to quarrel in public. In fact I did not mean to let myself go so far.

It seems to me that this letter recognises, more than any other which I have quoted, the underlying friction which permeated the medical staff. In one of the earliest chapters I wrote that my Father never talked much about his time in Russia and when I had almost completed my manuscript, I received a letter from Dr Michael Jefferson (he who was born in Petrograd at Christmas time 1916) using almost identical phraseology concerning his father. What

Fleming and Waterhouse thought I do not know, but Marshall (I am told) was silent as well. I have to suppose that all of them had a sense of disappointment about the whole enterprise.

I cannot conclude this chapter without offering some personal comments upon Father's letters. It is not possible to pretend that they were happy; in fact a general gloom pervades them I would say. 'I sometimes wonder if I shall ever be in the train for England' and 'We are living in a very depressing age and it is difficult to be cheerful'. Curiously, these Russian letters echo those which he had written four years earlier from America, whither he had gone for a tour of hospitals in the USA and Canada with a group of surgical colleagues from St Bartholomew's Hospital. I find almost the same remarks in both: 'I rather wish we had never come'; and 'We are really wasting our time'; and yet again, 'In spite of it all I am really homesick and wish you were here'.

That was the truth. He hated being separated from my mother, whom he addressed as Mittie or Mit (her given name was May) or 'Mim', a pleasing matronym which was invented by my brother Richard when he was about five years of age and which stuck to her for the rest of her life. All these names are to be found in his letters, together with those more affectionate terms which any man uses. His love-letters were couched in emotional words more appropriate, it might seem, for a young man in his twenties than for one in his forties. They recalled his courtship, the evening on which he proposed (though he is silent about his acceptance) and some wonderful occasions and nostalgic dinner parties. Constantly he wrote of Mim's beauty and indeed she was beautiful in the classical mould. As well, she had an attractive soprano voice, trained in Leipzig where she went as a girl to study singing under Richard Strauss and who was wont to refer to her as *mein kleiner Kanarianvogel.*

More than anything else perhaps, Father's letters looked forward to better times — 'let's go up to Scotland for a week's fishing' — and to the secure and happy family life which his whole upbringing demanded. Inevitably there were occasions when he was beset by doubts: 'I suppose one ought to be broadminded and allow one's wife to have her freedom during an enforced absence like this. Is it fair to expect she will not have some sort of fling if she is deserted for a year? I get fairly desperate and imagine all sorts of things . . .'

He had no need to. To the reassurance which he received, he replied:

So you think that a good many people have lost their heads because of the War. What 'goings-on' have you heard of lately? It is always interesting to hear of other peoples', though I don't allow it in my own family: which please to remember well.

On learning that Mim's sister-in-law had been delivered of a girl, he wrote: 'I am very envious, you can tell her. I wish I had a daughter: I live in hopes'. (Such hopes were not realised, which is scarcely surprising since my mother was 44 by the time he returned from Russia. Nevertheless I fear that, in this respect at least, I was a disappointment to him.) But he admitted compensations: 'I'm glad you have some children to worry about. They are interesting brats as was only to be expected with a mother of such striking individuality. My chief thought in life is when I shall see you again'.

I would have liked to have been able to record some shafts of humour in Father's letters, for he possessed a fine dry wit as I remember. There is none, unless one may include an observation that 'in many of the Bath Establishments they ask if you want a masseuse or a *femme* at 2, 3 or 4 Roubles according to choice', and one other story which is worth quoting. It came from the Berlitz School where he and his colleagues were doing their best to learn Russian and French.

The Frenchman at Berlitz told me yesterday about the young man who had just got married and telegraphed his mother-in-law: '7 et 3, 13 et 3' and received the reply: '6, 7 et 3; 7, 9'.

This may perhaps be transliterated *'C'est étroit, très étroit'* (and the reply) *'si c'est étroit, c'est neuf!'.* A French medical colleague tells me that there are many such mathematical jokes, some of which require a knowledge of quadratic equations for their solution! I think that Gibbon might approve my following his own practice of leaving such remarks 'in the decent obscurity of a learned tongue'.

His last letter from Petrograd, number 54, was dated October 8/21 1916.

My dearest Mim
. . . I expect to be home before this letter arrives. The weather here is appalling — snow, thaw, slush and as cold as the dickens. It is impossible to write as people come and interrupt me continually. As I shall come and tell you these things myself it is unnecessary to tell you that I love you.
Your devoted Douglas.

Father did not regret his departure. Fleming and Waterhouse had gone and he really wasn't too fond of Flavelle. Thompson, Jefferson and Marshall were only 'young lads': moreover there was a moratorium on doctors leaving England and he felt that if he did not get home then he never would. His admiration for the two Ladies was immense but his friendship with them was never more than formal I would say. He enjoyed his time in the Field more than at Base for, although at the Front the wounds were more horrifying, he felt that he was doing more useful and interesting work. In addition he could make his own decisions and, to use his own phrase, there was far less 'argyfying' at the Front.

So he leaves my stage, to return to Bart's and the 1st London General for the rest of the war. And after this interlude I myself return to tell of the fortunes of the hospital during its second year of life and death.

Decline and Exodus

I must say our medical and surgical staff for ability cannot be compared with that of last year.

[Lady Sybil to Lady Muriel. 31st January 1917.]

When WDH left for home in late October 1916 the writing was on the wall. Indeed it had been so for a long time because one of the earliest entries in his diary, at the time when he was trying to learn Russian at the Berlitz School, reads: 'The Frenchman at Berlitz says that the Govt. have moved their treasury to Novi Novgorod & that the Germans will be in Petrograd in Spring. *Nous verrons!*' Reading Pares's *Russian Memoirs* one gets the same impression of the failing competence of the government and the widespread feeling that it was only a matter of time before the whole country collapsed in revolution. To say the least the Army Directorate was uncertain and the Tsar himself had assumed the office of Commander-in-Chief 'because he believed he had a religious call to do so', having unwisely agreed to sack the Grand Duke Nicholas Nicoliaievich in September 1915 and who by general consent was pretty good at his job.

Behind everything brooded the sinister Rasputin: neither priest nor monk, but one of those *stranniki* or 'wanderers', whom Russian history has thrown up from time to time over the centuries. By birth Grigory Novykh, he acquired the nickname Rasputin, meaning dissolute or 'the debauchee' in his vicious youth and he certainly lived up to this reputation in later years.[1] How he obtained his influence over the Tsarina by claiming to be able to cure the haemophyllic heir to the throne, Alexis Nikolayievich, is well known. As Bernard Pares put it: 'Here is the great Orthodox Church with its gorgeous ceremonial and music, represented by a filthy lay-brother, a charlatan and adventurer'.

---

[1] Rasputin had the good fortune (if that is the appropriate phrase) to profess the belief that one could only attain redemption through sin.

On the night of 29th-30th December (16th-17th December OS) 1916, his planned assassination took place — though only just. The conspirators were Prince Felks Yusupov, a relation by marriage of the Tsar; the Grand Duke Dmitri, Vladimir Purishkevich, a member of the Duma (or Parliament); and a Doctor Lazovert, whose duty it was to prepare the poison for the cakes and wine which Rasputin was to be given at the midnight supper-party in the basement dining-room of Prince Yusupov's Palace on the Moika. He ate and drank and failed to die; and in a panic was shot three times at short range, first in the dining-room and then in the courtyard outside, by Yusupov and Purishkevich. Even that proved insufficient and he was finally dumped into the River Neva through a hole in the ice where he died. The post-mortem recorded death by drowning and that in spite of the presence of three bullet wounds; one in the chest 'which was mortal', one in the back, and one in the forehead 'which was discoloured by the powder'. It has always been a matter for argument whether Dr Lazovert lost his nerve and failed to produce the poison — or not enough of it, or whether Rasputin ate the wrong cakes. By order of the Tsarina he was embalmed and buried at Tsarskoe Selo. Two months later the body, 'looking as if it was still alive', was dug up by revolutionary soldiers, stripped and insulted and burnt at Udinli, 15 miles north of Petrograd.[2]

Prince Yusupov and Dmitri found sanctuary in the latter's Palace and here in due course they were sought by the supporters of Rasputin on the pretext of visiting some wounded patients. Lady Sybil Grey confronted them and refused them admission to *her hospital*. Like everyone else in Petrograd she was well aware that Yusupov was the murderer and wrote, 'there was an uproar of excitement and thankfulness, workers toasting him, nuns blessing him'. Only the Tsarina dissented. The Prince was arrested at the railway station on his way to the Crimea, the Duke ordered not to leave his Palace. There were rumours that both were to be executed 'causing great agitation among the factory workers: telephones (in the hospital) ringing all day to say that they had decided to form a body-guard to protect Yousoupoff'. Finally, to add a bizarre note to a situation which might even shake the sangfroid of a Hospital Administrator to-day: 'Y. got a fish-bone in his throat'. I wish I could add that WDH removed it, but of course

[2] See: *The Russian Diary of an Englishman* (William Heinemann, 1919) and *Rasputin* by Prince Yousoupoff [English translation by Oswald Rayner] (Jonathen Cape, 1927).

he was not longer there. In fact it was removed by Mr Geoffrey Jefferson.

'The Emperor returned from the Front (wrote Lady Sybil): his cheerfulness struck all those about him!' Trustworthy guards were placed at all the Palace (hospital) entrances and things calmed down. The Grand Duke Dmitri was ordered by the Tsar to attend his furthest estates in Persia and there we have news of him some months later 'kicking his heels, poor boy, in a rotten climate and very unhappy I believe'. Another source records that he was helpless and desolate and that following the murder he had *une crise de nerfs* and completely broke down in the train on his way to Persia. At least, in his isolation, he was relatively free from being himself assassinated.

It is difficult to exaggerate Lady Sybil's personal bravery on this occasion although in fact this was to be taxed to an equal extent a couple of months later. She alone held the key to the door of the private apartments which opened out of the entrance hall at the foot of the Great Staircase — a key 'of immense size', and this she wore round her neck and concealed in her corsage. However, like all proper palaces, there was a secret stairway which led from these apartments to an upper floor (this actually opened into the doctors' quarters) and it was by this means that the Grand Duke came and went until his banishment.

Lady Sybil recorded her own version of these stirring times in a letter to her brother-in-law, Evelyn Jones:

> Dear Jonah,   Jan. 1/14 1917
> I wouldn't be out of Russia for anything now. It is curious isn't it that things of immense moment and importance can only be accomplished by intrigue and murder. Can you imagine Tecks, Connaughts etc. doing the like in England? But the funny thing is that here one fits into the atmosphere to such an extent that one realises that it was the only thing to be done and that it was right and one thoroughly approves of the thing itself although perhaps not of the way it was carried out.

In this same letter there follow some stories about Rasputin and his astonishing power over men and women, particularly women. Thus:

> Here is one story which utterly passes my comprehension. I know you won't believe it but it's gospel truth. I heard it from a woman whom I absolutely trust, who saw it with her own eyes.

At dinner R. tearing the meat with his fingers an hands — dirty pig — and then the ladies (!!) licking his fingers afterwards. What was this curious fascination and hypnotism that he had over women that made them do such utterly revolting things? Most of the stories I couldn't possibly write. No — as the Russians say, we English out here even cannot understand to what extent they feel humiliated and to the same extent you cannot even understand what we feel.

In this same long letter there are two rather pleasant political 'asides', in keeping maybe with her Liberal upbringing. 'I hope the new Cabinet will be a success. Although L.G. is a liar etc. he certainly seems to be whole-hearted in ending the war victoriously. If we could have foreseen this five years ago what would we have said?' And again: 'Did you hear a nice little story about Asquith? Two days before he resigned he told a lady friend that he couldn't *possibly* resign because all the Stock Exchanges in the world would have a slump. Two days later stocks had gone up everywhere but the Mark had dropped. He then went to bed exceedingly ill!'

On 8th March 1917 there occurred the famous uprising in Petrograd. This has been documented many times, but since my own story is concerned more with the hospital than with the background of the event I will start by describing it in the words of one of the nurses who witnessed it.[3] I would remind the reader that the Dmitri Palace was situated on the Nevsky Prospekt and at the southern end of the Anichkov Bridge which spanned the Fontanka Canal, a sort of focal point for 'demos' in modern terminology. It was as if columns of marchers were converging upon Parliament Square from along the Strand and across Westminster Bridge.

On Friday March 9th things seemed to come to a climax. Cossacks kept riding up and down trying to disperse the crowd. Our hospital was given a guard of 30 soldiers, three of whom were on duty in the hall with fixed bayonets. Next day, from the hospital windows we had a splendid view of what took place on the Nevsky and watched what were probably the first shots fired, several people being hit. It seemed uncalled-for and brutal,

[3] The Russian Revolution seen from a Hospital Window. 'V.A.D.' *The Red Cross*. Vol. IV. 8. 15th August 1917.

as the crowd was thoroughly good tempered and talked and joked with the soldiers, who though ordered many times to fire, refused to do so.

On Sunday morning things seemed quieter; but the Russian rises late and it would take more than a Revolution to make the curious, who swell the crowd, rise early! Suddenly firing started. Ten wounded were brought to us, three already dead or dying on their stretchers. During the night . . . many regiments revolted, killing all the officers who refused to join them.

'VAD' and her colleagues had an exciting time getting back to the Nurses Home that night, escorted by two doctors and during a lull in the firing. 'We finally made a dash for our doorway across the street, the bullets throwing up a little shower of snow as they hit the pavement, but we all arrived safely.' They had a most disturbed night, the noise was terrific, people yelling and screaming, incessant firing. An angry mob demanded to search the building for hidden police and machine guns but the *sanitars* held them off successfully, saying it was a house for English Sisters. At the same time General Leman, in command of the Palace, interviewed the leaders of the mob, who claimed that there was a machine-gun on the roof and convinced them that it was an English hospital for Russian soldiers. He asked them to search quietly and not to alarm the patients. This seemed to satisfy them and they left — after first removing the General's sword.

The rioting continued for some ten days, with battles here and there. Food was scarce; black bread only. The nurse's account concludes:

Everywhere people were busy tearing down Imperial emblems, all the Eagles being hastily removed from shops under Royal patronage. Our Palace Eagle met its end, a heap of plaster on the road it had proudly gazed on for many years.

Bernard Pares was also at the hospital during this week; and at some personal risk he addressed the crowds (since he spoke Russian fluently) advising them on the merits of the alliance with Britain and against the propaganda of the Leninists. Late one night he found it advisable to seek sanctuary in the porch of the British Embassy which was also on the Nevsky. Finding to his surprise that the door was unlocked, he went into the hall and discovered, to his greater surprise and even alarm, that the solitary guard was asleep. He went upstairs, knocked on Sir George's bedroom door and waking him from sleep, suggested that there should perhaps be a somewhat higher degree of security.

Lady Sybil too recorded her impressions of these few momentous and frightening days. Although she had the Russian General Leman at her side, as the official Commander of the hospital, both she and he were very much at risk. It should be emphasised that the British and particularly the Ambassador, Sir George Buchanan, were extremely popular in Petrograd at this time and he wisely advised her to make the most of this fact. Consequently: 'we made as many Red Cross flags as we could and hung a very big Union Jack from the balcony. We made them out of old sheets and an old Father Christmas coat. Three flags were stolen as soon as put up; feverish haste to make more. Should we use red bed-jackets?'

The night of the 12th-13th March was particularly bad. An hotel next to the Nurses Home was sacked and many of the police, whose headquarters it was, were murdered. 'The Staff at the Club had a terrible time.' Then at 11.30 p.m., as Lady Sybil was doing her Night Round of the wards, four soldiers with fixed bayonets came in, officered by a young student carrying a revolver who '. . . pointing it at my chest started a speech in Russian which I understood enough to realise he was talking about wine; and felt it prudent to offer him all we had. I then found to my amusement that he was offering *us* wine at the point of the revolver as Kerensky had ordered all wine cellars to be emptied and the wine given to the hospitals in order to prevent drunkeness'.

The staff slept in their clothes that night. The next morning the Astoria Hotel was attacked by a howling, raging mob armed to the teeth, who sacked the ground floor (for the hotel was an Allied Head-quarters), killed the Russian officers and surged up the staircase shooting in all directions. The British officers naturally thought that their last moment had come, particularly as many of the mob were drunk and by this time many criminals, released from the prisons, were among them. To their amazement (wrote Lady Sybil) the moment the crowd saw English uniforms they stopped. Some even took off their hats and said: 'English officers, forgive us, we do not wish to bother you' and passed on in the most courteous manner possible to do more destruction . . .

The next day was more peaceful and by 9 p.m. the shooting had more or less ceased. However at 11.30 p.m. 'I had just got all Sisters settled for the night when three drunken soldiers came into the

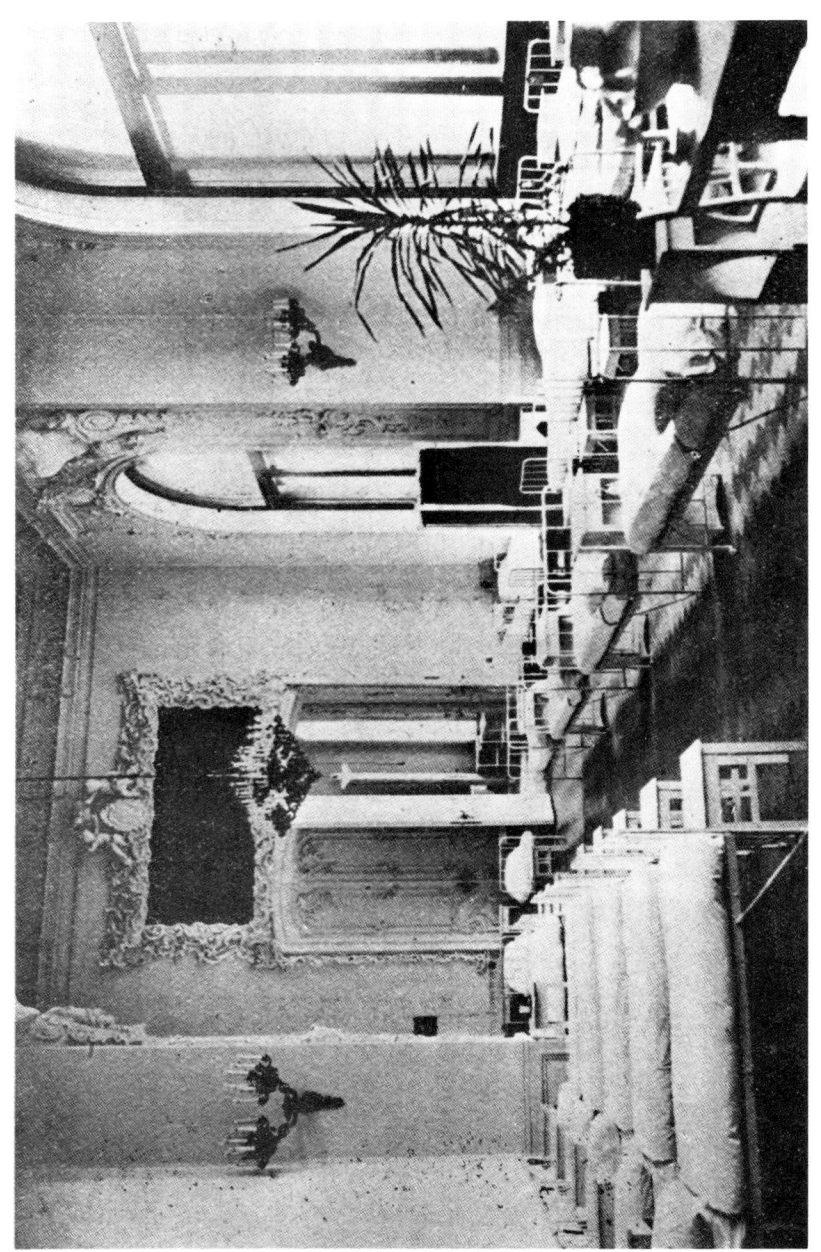

A WARD IN THE HOSPITAL

hospital brandishing naked swords and one with a loaded rifle wanting his finger bandaged. They were quite amiable and we were very nice and civil to them.' Later: 'very heavy firing. Bullet through window of Ward C high up. Patients panicky'.

The hospital had guards, from the Siniowski regiment, but they soon decamped to join the revolutionaires. 'Mr Garstin (from the Embassy) telephoned at 3 a.m. Impossible to find other guards. He advised us to hang out a bigger Union Jack so I hung it on the inside of the stairs.' Later on that dreadful night 16 men arrived and demanded 25 suits of underlinen for their soldiers. When asked for his authority the officer, looking most insolent, replied: 'It is not a request — it is a command'. Sixteen bayonets won the day, was Lady Sybil's laconic comment.

On Friday, 16th March (3rd March OS) Lady Sybil recorded two events which are so strikingly inconsequent that they are worth recording as she wrote them down at the time. The first:

> The Emperor has abdicated — and his son. Also the Grand Duke Michael. The Revolutionary flag has been hoisted on the Winter Palace. All crowns — double eagles — and Imperial cyphers were hastily torn down and thrown into the canals. Only the eagles on the Emperor's huge Winter Palace were left and draped in red. *Rumours.* The Grand Duke has died of measles. There has been a three-day revolution in Berlin. The Kaiser is a prisoner. The Crown Prince is killed. The Germans have taken Riga.
> *Facts.* Heavy snowstorms and many carts of provisions. People happier.

and the second:

> Dr. Flavelle, Head of Field Hospital, arrived at 3 am having heard nothing of any trouble until within fifty versts of Petrograd!

The observation made by Lady Sybil which heads this chapter was unfortunately true. She may perhaps have had in mind the Russian proverb, 'Praise the cow and she will withhold her milk'; but from the start the replacement of staff had been a difficulty and by 1917 the demands of the Western Front had made things even more difficult, both on the medical and nursing sides. Waterhouse and WDH, the chief surgeons, had gone and so had Fleming, who at any rate had been able to deputise for them. Jefferson, who did so well at Lutsk in the summer and autumn of '16 had held the fort in Petrograd during the winter months. But Lady Sybil quite properly had to think of the coming year of '17 and of what might be required. WDH himself had anticipated this when, longing to get home, he had written to my mother: 'If you hear of anybody who would be prepared to take my place, please let me know'. At one point it was thought that Mr James Berry, the Royal Free Hospital surgeon who had done splendid work for the Red Cross in Serbia, might be prepared to take his place, 'but (the letter continues) Berry says he will only come if he can bring Mrs. B. with him and that isn't very popular with the authorities out here I'm afraid'. Actually, WDH's letters make several references to the possibility of my mother joining him in Petrograd but quite apart from the difficulty of leaving three young children behind in England, it never really seemed likely.

One member of the staff managed to achieve this — or to be more accurate, his wife did. Mrs Jefferson, herself a qualified doctor, through family connexions knew the Canadian High Commissioner in London. By 'feminine wiles' she managed to reach Petrograd without even her husband's knowledge and for some time served with a medical unit near the Austrian frontier. Mr Jefferson's gratification at her arrival was doubtless increased by the fact that just before Christmas she gave birth to a son who was able to attend the New Year party at the hospital at the age of three weeks — 'the smallest thing I have ever seen', as Lady Sybil remarked. This son become Dr Michael Jefferson DM, FRCP, who tells me that he is not altogether surprised at Lady Sybil's observation since he was born eight weeks prematurely.

About this time Lady Sybil must have been feeling very much alone. She had recently received a letter of immense length and much consequence from Lady Muriel in London who was clearly equally worried about their beloved hospital. I quote from it *in extenso* but because much of it was obviously confidential I have considered it proper to suppress some of the names mentioned.

Dearest Sybil

This week has been a terrible rush, hospital and kitchen work . . . I am going to Cranmore until January 9th but have arranged everything . . . Can you get the men employment in Kieff to keep them out of mischief, either as orderlies or drivers if they are obliged to be there? — they are all men who want to be kept at work! I expect you heard the excitement about D—. Neither Lord L. nor any member of the Com. have ever heard of him let alone seen him so he lied deliberately on that subject. He was sore at not being put in charge of the Motor Column but as he understood nothing about management of men, driving or machinery there was never a question of this. In fact I never saw a more miserable collection of men than were sent out. I have heard of excellent men over here who could have come and can't think why no responsible people in the motor line were approached. Most of them treated their agreement as a Cook's Touring ticket to Russia and were extraordinarily inefficient.

Now a very happy Christmas which I know you will have because you will like making everyone have a good time in the hospital[4]— please give them all many greetings from me . . .

Lady Muriel then passed, in her general review, to the medical staff:

When I came out last year I had a very difficult time from the moment I arrived. As you know there was almost mutiny amongst the medical staff and a certain amount of dissatisfaction among the nursing staff and very general outside criticism. I was told certain things that can't be repeated that confirmed my suspicions in certain directions. Then added to this our surgeons were replaced by physicians which did not assist the smooth running of a surgical hospital! With all these difficulties to face and no strong man as C.O., in fact practically no C.O. at all, the only thing was to make the best of things all round till better conditions prevailed.

Dr.— has proved a real rotter. He wrote to the War Office that our hospital was not wanted and that young men like Jefferson and Marshall should be recalled as their work could equally well be done by older & less efficient men. This was sent to Lord Cheylesmore who played up well and [said that] if a man was so disloyal it would not be well to employ him on the W.O. staff. G— seems to have talked in this way too: however what

---

[4] They did, too: Salmon, turkey, rich and very good plum puddings. Lady Sybil 'found some dear little white Ensigns and had Anglo-Russian Hospital Xmas 1916 printed on them in gold in one corner and one stood up in each napkin at each place. Forty-nine was the number that sat down. We did two plays: the first is not very good — it is acted by Doctor Williams who thinks himself an Irving and is really a stick. Miss Curtis and Miss Jameson excellent. The other play is called 'The Rest Cure' — v. amusing, all about a nursing home and it takes off the nursing profession. Mr Jefferson acts the nervous patient quite admirably: it is very funny'.

does anything matter and none of these men count a d— as long as the work is well done by those on the spot and I do feel all the rotters have gone now and it must be a pleasant change to feel there is no intriguing etc. I hear Dr. May says that Harmer ought to have left in May but where should we have been without him when he nobly stepped *(sic)* into the hole made by May and Gardner.

Hugh Walpole, recently returned from Petrograd, had apparently been to see Lady Muriel and informed her of considerable anti-British and pro-German feeling in Russia 'some of which has penetrated into the bureau with reference to our hospital'. The letter continues:

> I knew all the time that certain agents were savage at any success we had. I told Mr. Walpole several facts which seemed to be new to him? . . .
>
> Mr. Walpole was altogether rather nervous about you and me and seemed to think that we were like a Seidlitz powder and that our views never coincide. I pointed out that if this were so, we should not be working together now because it is impossible to run two policies — or two anythings — in an organisation like this. Unless there is very definite discipline the position is impossible and there was too much of everyone wanting to run the show in the beginning. I see no real point of difference between us but if you feel they exist as strongly as Mr. Walpole leads me to believe do tell me what they are. According to him Matron rather runs with the hare and hunts with the hounds — this I had been told before but would not believe and still doubt. You are bound to hear as many criticisms of my work as I heard of yours, people enjoy nothing more than repeating things generally . . . It is much better to ignore it. I am sure the chief source of this, however, has left! So tell me what you have at the back of your head, Sybil dear, and what your points of difference are so that there shall be no misunderstandings in a work about which there can be no two opinions can there?

There was a good deal more of this letter, for neither Lady Muriel nor Lady Sybil spared themselves when they put pen to paper, nine or ten quarto pages being by no means exceptional. To me it seems that this particular one was evidence of some sort of crisis between them and it recalls the *cri-de-coeur* of Churchill writing to Roosevelt: 'Anything like a real disagreement between us would break my heart'.

However it ended happily: 'Well, best of loves and I have a tiny present for you that will follow, also one for the Matron please tell her. Yours really affec. Muriel'. And then a postscript: 'This mostly written in train so please forgive scrawl'.

Lady Sybil's reply was both shorter and more factual:

> I expect Jefferson will remain. He is better up here [Petrograd] than at the Field, because he is a very good operator but *very* slow, which is quite a disadvantage in a Field Hospital.[5] Is Harmer coming out again? He is not such a strong and pig-headed man as Flavelle but he has 1000 times more tact, speaks French and understands a lot of Russian.

Things were obviously not easy. She still had Marshall of course and the young Thompson but locums came and went and she knew that this was no way to run a hospital. To add to her troubles, the excellent Miss Irvine Robertson had had to return to England at the end of January, protesting valiantly, because of her increasing arthritis.

It was an inauspicious start to a year which witnessed the decline and fall of the Russian Empire and as a very minor consequence, the decline and exodus of the Anglo-Russian Hospital.

The actual work of the hospitals during this year is not easy to determine though briefly it may be divided into what happened in Petrograd and the activities of the staff on the South-Western Front, in the Bukovina and in the Carpathians.

As to the first, the Dmitri Palace had a comparatively slack time, at any rate from the surgical point of view. Their extra-curricular activities were certainly exciting enough, for a Bolshevik rising had failed in Petrograd in July, being put down by the Cossack cavalry. Once again the Hospital had had a ringside seat of the activity, Lady Muriel enjoying it tremendously from an upper window 'though bullets were flying'. During this episode over 60 casualties, some civilian and some among the soldiery, were admitted to the hospital. Most of these patients were 'docile and sensible though there were a few born agitators'. With seething revolution the authorities were

---

[5] In this judgment she was remarkably perceptive. As already noted, Jefferson was to become one of the world's leading neurosurgeons: and anyone who has had any experience of that particular speciality will be familiar with the meticulous care and total disregard for the passage of time which an operation on the brain may involve, four or five hours being more or less routine.

anxious to keep the wounded away from Petrograd. Consequently the beds were filled with medical patients and the staff saw many cases of an unaccustomed disease, scurvy, mainly from the Northern Front where food was desperately scarce. A most interesting sidelight on this matter came to light among Sir Geoffrey Jefferson's papers, in the form of a pencilled 'Account' which he wrote after his return to Petrograd from the Southern Front. 'Since the days of The Great Retreat in 1915 (he wrote) there have never been a great number of wounded coming to Petrograd. It lies too far north of the line [patients took 4-7 days to come from Dvinsk and Riga] for us to receive large convoys. But for the amount of valuable time and money that had been spent on making the Dmitri Palace as excellent a hospital as it undoubtedly is, and the vast expense of transferring and refitting in some town further south such as Kiev, I feel sure we should have pressed for a move.' Here was unexpected confirmation of that entry in WDH's diary, already quoted: 'Lady M. back again. Talked all day about what to do. She wants to move to Kieff.'

The English Diarist had recorded at about this time that 'things go from worse to worst. God alone knows what will happen'; and about this time also Fleming and Jefferson were preparing the Report (which has been mentioned in chapter 9) explaining a situation which must have made strange reading to those in England who knew how a hospital should be conducted.

> Our *sanitars* were loyal to us — barring their decision to plan and control their own work. But the old feeling of security, the feeling that an order given, however necessary and reasonable, might not be carried out unless the recipient of the order felt that his own convenience and dignity were not impeached by it, had passed away. One must experience a revolution . . . to realise the absolute impotence of the individual. All authority goes, there is no one to back one up . . . In a foreign land with a strange tongue the difficulties are enormously enhanced.

Perhaps Lady Muriel, with her favourite remark, 'Rubbish! What is all the fuss about?' might have overcome such insubordination, but she did not get back to Russia until the end of May, having been kept in England organising the A-R H. Exhibition at the Grafton Galleries. The month of June 1917 must have been one of the few occasions when she and Lady Sybil were in the same place and at the same time. Before long Lady Muriel went south to oversee the field hospital and

128

the motor column but Lady Sybil's tenure of the base hospital was unhappily cut short by the news that her father was suffering from a mortal illness and she had to return to England. Earl Grey died at the end of August and Lady Sybil never again returned to Russia.

The field hospital had a more active time and before long was to enjoy what may have been its finest hour. With the summer thaw General Brusilov had staged an advance around Minsk and there was great rejoicing that the Germans were about to be defeated. Jefferson wrote: 'Brusilov is a born fighter and hates inactivity'; and he went on; 'war on the Russian Front is in many ways a more human affair than it is in France. There is less marching, more movement and more open fighting. At heart the Russian despises trench warfare and never takes the trouble over his trenches that the Austrian does. Of course all this in modern warefare spells casualties and certainly our field units never suffered from lack of material. At times we were extraordinarily hard-pressed and our accommodation pressed to the limit. Room had to be found by pushing two beds together and laying three people on the two beds crosswise and so on'.

Now Lady Muriel went to Kiev and from there to Czernowitz to join the field hospital. The situation displeased her.

> Found that the new head of the hospital appointed by the soldiers' and workmen's committee was a woman spy. Recognised by a nurse, trying to get into the hospital. Two revolvers found in skirtband. Then bombed . . . so we evacuated. Left at four in the morning. Kitten lost, so start postponed for an hour till found.

From there to Kamenets Podolsk, which reminded both her and Sister Mavor of St Andrews in Scotland, not least because the latter had been Matron of the City Hospital in that town before going to Russia. Theirs was the only hospital unit equipped for surgical work and in ten days they treated 5000 wounded, many of whom (she noted) had their left hands shot off. 'They put a loaf of bread on the muzzle of the rifle and their left hand on top of it, and then fire, so that they should not have to go back to the Front. It was horrible . . .'

Once again they were ordered to retreat, though Lady Muriel at first refused. They crossed into Roumania, to Dorohiou (or Dorohoi) where they commandeered a school. The Mayor of the village was loud in his praise and admiration for the British. Here they remained for some time but Lady Muriel, visiting Kiev for supplies, contracted typhoid fever, of which there was an epidemic at that time. She was taken back to Petrograd in a derelict car with no brakes — a hazardous journey — and for several weeks was a desperately ill patient in her own hospital. Discipline was very poor (as Lord Cheylesmore reported) and the male *sanitars* had been replaced by women, 'simple peasants who . . . goggled at the miracle of modern science and who crossed themselves devoutly when for the first time they saw water running from a tap'.[6]

From her sick-bed she had sharp battles with the medical staff and the formidable Lady Georgina. But Sir George remained her friend. 'He presented me with my medal (the OBE) on Sunday & was very nice. It is an ugly thing & I am sorry it will circulate widely among foreigners: our medals have not been so bad up till now.'

Of the activities of the motor column during these few months I have been unable to find many details. It may be assumed that they were ferrying the wounded over the 'corduroy' roads between the Fronts and the nearest hospitals. But these Fronts were in a constant state of flux and little by little the superior German efficiency was pushing them back. Halicz, Ternopol, Stanislav and Czernowitz fell in turn during July and August: and in the north, Riga — the gateway to Petrograd — succumbed quite suddenly in September. The war in the East was virtually over but for political purposes alone the Western Allies were concerned to keep the Russians in the field. What is certain is that the field hospital and the motor column slowly retreated through Bessarabia and found their last home in Odessa on the Black Sea.

Shortly after the Tsar abdicated in March 1917 a Provisional Government under Prince Lvov had been set up. The threat from the Bolsheviks, still mostly in hiding or, like Lenin and his colleagues, in exile in Switzerland, seemed to have been set aside. But with the publication of *Army Order Number One*, which abolished the military salute to officers and virtually put an end to any sort of discipline, the floodgates were opened. There were said to be two million deserters.

---

[6] It is easy to feel smug about such conditions existing in 1917. But Dr C. B. Lewis, my friend and anaesthetist at the Royal Marsden Hospital in London for 20 years, and who was serving with the RAMC in 1945 when the British and Russian armies made contact in Germany, has told me that a number of Russian wounded in his hospital spent many happy hours flushing the lavatories because they had never before seen such things.

It was in April that Lenin arrived in Petrograd preaching the new dogma, but this took the best part of three months to reach the armies on the Southern Front. Bernard Pares, who was then with Kebel helping to organise the motor column in the Bukovina, had of course seen it coming for over a year and had so advised the Foreign Office. Now Miss Florence Farmborough, nursing with the Russian Red Cross on a neighbouring Front, was able to observe the system at close hand:

Saturday, 26th August 1917
We have been told that a meeting is to be held in the neighbourhood. Strange-looking men, some in uniform, others in civilian clothes have been organising informal meetings with the troops. So now that such a personage is due to visit our Front, we Sisters are extremely anxious to hear for ourselves the 'message of good will' which he is supposed to deliver.

Sunday, 27th August
It was a most extraordinary meeting! Never in our wildest dreams did we imagine that we should listen to such an outpouring of treachery.

The man who had come to speak to the soldiers had an ordinary face and was dressed in ordinary Russian clothes. He spoke for a time about Russia, her vast territory, her wealth and her overlords who, possessing enormous estates and resources were revered on account of their riches throughout the western world. Then he described the impoverished peasantry who, unschooled, uncared-for and half-starved, were eking out a miserable existance by tilling and cultivating the land belonging to those same overlords. War had burst upon Russia and enemies had invaded our territory, and who were the men who had sacrificed themselves to fight the ruthless invaders and drive them off Russian soil? Not the wealthy overlords not the despotic landowners; no! They were safely installed in their fortress-homes. It was those down-trodden countrymen who had been roped in in their thousands, in their millions, to stem the tide of invasion.

But now a miraculous event had taken place! The Tsar, that arch-potentate, that arch-tyrant — had been dethroned and dismissed. Russia had been pronounced a free country! Freedom had come at last to the down-trodden people of Russia.

But war was an enemy of freedom, because it destroyed peace, and without peace there could be no freedom. It was up to the Russian soldier to do all in his power to procure peace. And the best and quickest way to bring about a guaranteed peace was to refuse to fight. Then, when peace had at last come to Russia, freedom could be enjoyed. The free men of Free Russia would own their own land. The great tracts of privately-owned territory would be split up and divided fairly among the peasantry. There would be common ownership of all properties and possessions.

Without offering an opinion on the political propriety of such a liaison with Army HQ it may be stated with assurance that this was not the most satisfactory way of arresting the advances of the German and Austrian troops. The Front was in fact in chaos and the task of the field hospital became increasingly difficult. Central organisation had become almost impossible and one can read this in the letters which were passing between Petrograd and London at the time. One such letter shows how wrong an intelligent observer could be. Jefferson, to his wife: early in May 1917, from Petrograd.

> Quiet here now: lots of silly rumours. There is a socialist erratic called Lenin at large; came from Switzerland via *Germany* (mark you!) and is preaching Stop The War, and doing a lot of harm. To-day many of our wounded went in procession to the Duma, voted for the continuation of the war and the arrest of Lenin — which I hope will be a fait accompli within a few days.

And a week later:

> Just called to see a man shot in the ankle by one of the Lenin Stop The War gang. However I don't anticipate much trouble from them. They are very much outnumbered and even if they got the upper hand in Petrograd the rest of Russia wouldn't put up with it.

Nor was he the only one to be fooled. Almost two years later and after the Bolshevik Revolution, we find HM Consul-General for South Russia writing to Lady Muriel: 'Bolshevism is tottering to its fall. I do not vary the opinion I expressed some six weeks ago that Petrograd and Moscow will be freed from the Bolsheviks within the next 2-3 months'.

In what I have called the Report to the shareholders of the A-R H. Lord Cheylesmore had made this observation:

> The question of the withdrawal of the Hospital, under the conditions now prevailing in Russia, has been seriously considered by the Committee, but they have been advised that it should remain for the present as a practical demonstration of our desire to help our Ally.

The date at the foot of the Report was 28th November 1917 but this pious aspiration was not to be realised. Exactly six weeks later, on 18th January 1918 the third and last Commandant, Dr Walter Yeld, who subsequently enlisted in the Royal Navy, took the staff out of Petrograd and across the Finnish border. Almost the last authentic reference to the hospital is a letter sent by him from Stockholm (where his party had just missed a boat to England) to Lady Muriel, who he supposed to be in Odessa. He was clearly very concerned about her safety and also confused about the instructions which he had been receiving from London.

My dear Lady Muriel   Jan 18 1918.
We are now on our way home, going on to Christiania tonight. I suppose you will now be returning to Petrograd [but] I don't understand them first allowing and then disallowing your staying at Odessa. I wish you had returned at once and I feel worried about you. They have been pressing us very much from London to leave Petrograd and said there was no necessity to wait for you!

Dr Yeld's letter continues with details of the arrangements which he hoped he had made with the Russian Red Cross, itself in considerable disarray, for the stores and equipment of the Hospital. Finally he offered some practical advice: 'If you have any roubles get rid of them here! You can get about 100 Kroner for 150 roubles which means that £4 worth of roubles will get you £7 worth of Kroner. Don't forget when you travel!'

That Lady Muriel received this letter is evident from the fact that it is among her correspondence. It is also evident that she took not the slightest notice of it, as her future travels proved.

The BRCS Commissioner in Petrograd, Mr R. E. Kimens, had been pretty well at his wits end in attempting to keep the hospital in being. He had already notified the Committee in London of the chaos in Petrograd, the looting of stores and so on and had reported that 'I am extremely glad that the Society's units have left Russia: they are not wanted as there is no fighting at the Front'. Now he advised Lady Muriel, who was actually near Kiev and typically refusing to admit defeat:

British Embassy, Petrograd

Dear lady Muriel   25th January 1918

Your letter of January 7th reached me on the 21st inst. but I could not write sooner as I did not know of somebody going to Kieff. Following Dr. Yeld's departure on the 12th inst. the Hospital was handed over to the Russian Red Cross and four members, Mlle. Danzas, Col. Fenoult, Mr. Leech and myself were appointed by Dr. Yeld to look after the equipment and inventory which remains the property of the A.R.H. The Club at the Vladimirsky has been closed. All Russian nurses have left.

As you probably know the Red Cross in Petrograd has been seized by the Maximalist Government and Messrs. Petrovsky, Ordin and Czamansky are under arrest. [In answer to] the telegram I received from Lord Cheylesmore I replied that I could make no arrangements from here with regard to the return of the Unit in South Russia.

I am afraid it will be very difficult to send your personal luggage to Kieff owing to prevailing conditions . . .

And so that was the end of it. Lady Muriel got out of Kiev with the British Mission at the end of February, just in time before it was occupied by the Germans. Thence to Odessa, taking the rump of the A-R H. with her; but it was like the frying-pan and the fire, for there the Bolsheviks were in control and everything was in chaos. The British Consul Mr Picton Bagge (who oddly enough had been at King's College Cambridge a year after my father), found himself face to face with their Commander and was startled to recognise his partner in the previous year's tennis tournament in Odessa! Tactfully exploiting the situation he managed to arrange the evacuation of the A-R H. and other British nationals, a total of 40 persons, in an unsprung fourth-class railway carriage, padded for the transport of lunatics, to Moscow. There he hired two coaches on the Trans-Siberian express together with five Red Guards to preserve them from deserting soldiers; and these accompanied them as far as Irkutsk. Lady

Muriel, being more practical I would suppose, bought eight sucking pigs and a large quantity of black bread on the black market to sustain them for at least a part of their journey. Amongst the party were Sister Mary Macdonald, the photographer whom we met in chapter 4 and Sister Mavor; but there was also a more significant person — a Mr Thomas Marsden, as named on his passport. In reality this was Thomas Mazaryk, the Czech patriot who was to become the first President of the new state of Czechoslovakia.

As mentioned in an earlier chapter Lady Muriel was a great friend of Alice Mazaryk and it is likely that it was she who organised the passport for 'Mr Marsden'. Bagge did even better, for on his own authority he advanced Mazaryk £100,000 in Foreign Office bills to bring him and his army across Siberia and the Pacific Ocean to Vancouver, before repatriation to their homeland. The story of this incredible achievement is well known and certainly has no direct connexion with the Anglo-Russian Hospital, yet it has a bearing on Lady Muriel's future activities and therefore may be briefly recapitulated. Many Czechs had been enlisted in the Austro-Hungarian army but at the same time a corps of emigré Czechs and Slovaks had been serving with the Russians on the Southern Front. Prisoners-of-war increased in numbers and together with mass desertions, the corps had swelled into an army of some 60,000 troops. Mazaryk got them home.

Following the Treaty of Versailles, the revision of frontiers in Central Europe had created areas in Slovakia where food shortage was widespread and intense, the main victims being children suffering from severe malnutrition. Lady Muriel's instant response from Alice Mazaryk was to recruit a team of qualified welfare workers and to transport them to Slovakia as 'The Paget Mission'. Their uniform she designed herself and it is wearing this that she is illustrated on page 13. She established clinics in crisis areas and trained Czechoslovak women to carry on the work when the Mission returned to England.

It remains to summarise the journey (which is described by Blunt in detail in *Lady Muriel*). From Vladisvostock they went to Kyoto and there the Japanese Red Cross presented her with the Nightingale Medal, depicting a charming little enamelled bird and which was awarded annually 'To the Nurse who works not only with her Head but with her Heart'. Thence to San Francisco and Washington, where she had the honour of being received by the President himself; and it would seem, to considerable effect. There is the testimony of an American friend 'Olga' who wrote to her:

It is being said by *everyone* in Washington that your talk with Wilson had done more to influence him on the Russian situation than anything or anyone he has talked to before. I heard this straight from 'official circles' and was so thrilled that I *had* to let you know about it.

Lady Muriel remained in Washington for two weeks and to her surprise received a telegram from Sir Richard who was in New York on Admiralty business at that time. From New York she moved to Toronto and Montreal before setting sail for home.

Her party arrived in Liverpool on 26th May, nearly three months after leaving Kiev.

Materia Medica

During the 11 months between November 1915 and October 1916 more than 6,000 patients received treatment in the Anglo-Russian Hospitals. This was as nothing compared with the actual casualties on either the Eastern or Western Fronts during that same year. But numbers are not everything; and the hospitals did excellent work and made some interesting observations concerning the different sorts of injuries and their effects, sustained on these two Fronts. It was possible to draw some conclusions regarding comparative methods of treatment for infected wounds and these were published the following year.[1] The authors would have wished to have done better but as the introduction to their paper states, practically all their medical notes and records were confiscated at the frontier 'owing to the stupidity of a Russian Customs Official, who in spite of our strenuous protest, couched in very indifferent Russian, tore up the manuscripts under the notion that they contained treasonable matter'. Mr Marshall was more fortunate when he returned some months later and was able to bring home some of his own material. Perhaps this explains the paucity of medical information about the hospital, for apart from Mr Jefferson's paper in the *British Journal of Surgery*, which recorded the removal of a bullet from a soldier's cerebellum,[2] I can find none other. The contrast with the literature published from the Western Front is most marked.

Two of the most terrible scourges afflicting the wounded on the battlefields were tetanus and gas-gangrene. Sulphonamides and anti-biotics were as yet undiscovered and even the available anti-sera were unreliable. Antiseptics were therefore the main hope of saving lives and limbs, apart of course from whatever surgery was necessary. At this time several new antiseptics were under trial and some older ones were being rejected. The surgeons 'unhesitatingly condemned' pure

[1] *British Medical Journal: Notes from the Anglo-Russian Hospitals.* 6th October 1917. Sir Herbert F. Waterhouse FRCS, W. Douglas Harmer MC(Cantab), FRCS, Charles J. Marshall MS, FRCS.

[2] *British Journal of Surgery:* Vol. 5, 1918.

carbolic acid but thought very highly of Eusol (the Edinburgh University Solution) invented by Professor Loraine Smith and the hypertonic saline solution of Sir Almroth Wright. 'We treated hundreds of infected wounds and infected compound fractures with both of these but are not yet convinced which method presents the greater advantages. We can only state that both are, in our opinion, a great advance on older methods of treatment.' On the Western Front that superb surgeon, Gordon Taylor found the same. He became a leading authority on war wounds, writing at least 14 papers on this subject. In 1939 when war was once again inevitable he wrote *The Abdominal Injuries of Warfare,* a solemn preparation for the younger surgeons who would shortly have to deal with these. He dedicated this book to 'The Casualty Clearing Surgeons of the Franco-British Western Front 1914-1918' and being a scholar as well as a surgeon, he inscribed the title-page with a quotation from Lucan's *Pharsalia:*

> *. . . quid in arma furentem*
> *Impulerit populum, quid pacem excusserit orbi.*[3]

But to return to the more mundane matter of antiseptics. In the absence of anti-tetanic serum, extensive wounds were 'freely opened and finely powdered potassium permanganate (about 1 oz.) rubbed into all surfaces'. The wound 'smoked and assumed a blackened appearance', which may today sound pretty horrifying, but 'in hundreds of cases of infected wounds (including compound fractures) it was attended with the happiest results'. Another life-saving therapy in many apparently hopeless cases of septicaemia and pyaemia was the intravenous injection of Eusol solution, 100 cc. being given daily for several days. No toxic symptoms were ever observed, but the treatment was found to be ineffective for streptococcal, in distinction to other bacterial infections. There was also BIPP (Bismuth-iodoform-paraffin-paste) invented by Professor Rutherford Morison, which proved quite excellent for packing extensive gunshot wounds, preventing secondary infection and assisting the natural healing process.

---

[3] For those less well endowed, Sir Edward Ridley's translation must suffice:

> Why did a maddened people rush to arms
> And rob the world of peace.

Sir Gordon Gordon-Taylor KBE, CB, LLD and Fellow of four Colleges of Surgeons had the unusual distinction of being a Major-General in WWI. and a Rear-Admiral in WWII. The 'best loved surgeon in the world', he died aged 82 after being knocked down by a taxi when leaving Lord's Cricket Ground.

Iodoform poisoning was seldom if ever found, though occasionally dermatitis of the surrounding skin occurred.

There were some interesting and surprising differences observed between wounds sustained in Flanders and in Russia. Tetanus for example, so common in the former was almost unknown in the latter, only three cases being identified with certainty. Perhaps the appalling cold as well as the comparative lack of husbandry was responsible. On the other hand gas-gangrene was rife and responsible for the majority of deaths in the field hospitals — 'this terrible condition . . . with is vilely putrescent odour and grave toxaemic symptoms'. At one time Dr Rosher reported finding the bacillus in 80% of all the wounds from which he took cultures though this did not mean that the patients were suffering the disease in its clinical form. He concurred in the opinion of his surgical colleagues that the employment of Eusol, both locally and as an intravenous injection, was a most valuable phophylactic agent. Two things the surgeons learned about this infection. First, that the injection of hydrogen peroxide, a most powerful oxidising agent, into the affected tissues was not only useless but actually spread the disease by increasing the tension in the muscles involved. This treatment had been recommended on the theoretical basis that the anaerobic *Bacillus aerogenes capsulatus* (or *B. Welchii* as it was more commonly called) should be eliminated in a milieu of oxygen. It was not so. The second was that in order to save life, entire muscle-bundles from origin to insertion, had to be excised; or if this was impracticable, amputation became essential.

A rather remarkable case may be quoted: a Russian Colonel, who had been left for five days in the open after being wounded, was admitted with extensive gas-gangrene involving the whole of the upper extremity and spreading for several inches onto the chest wall. There seemed to be small hope of saving his life but 'as the patient's condition appeared desperate in the extreme, disarticulation at the shoulder-joint was performed and an intravenous injection of normal saline solution given on the operating table. Despite the extension of the gas-gangrene to the subcutaneous tissue of the chest, the patient made a rapid recovery'. That was the account published in the *British Medical Journal* 18 months after the event. But two other references to this fortunate Colonel are also on record. In a letter dated 14th August WDH wrote: 'We have had a lot of gas-gangrene which has meant amputations. One man — an officer — whose arm I took off at the shoulder has made a very remarkable recovery'. Lady Muriel was also

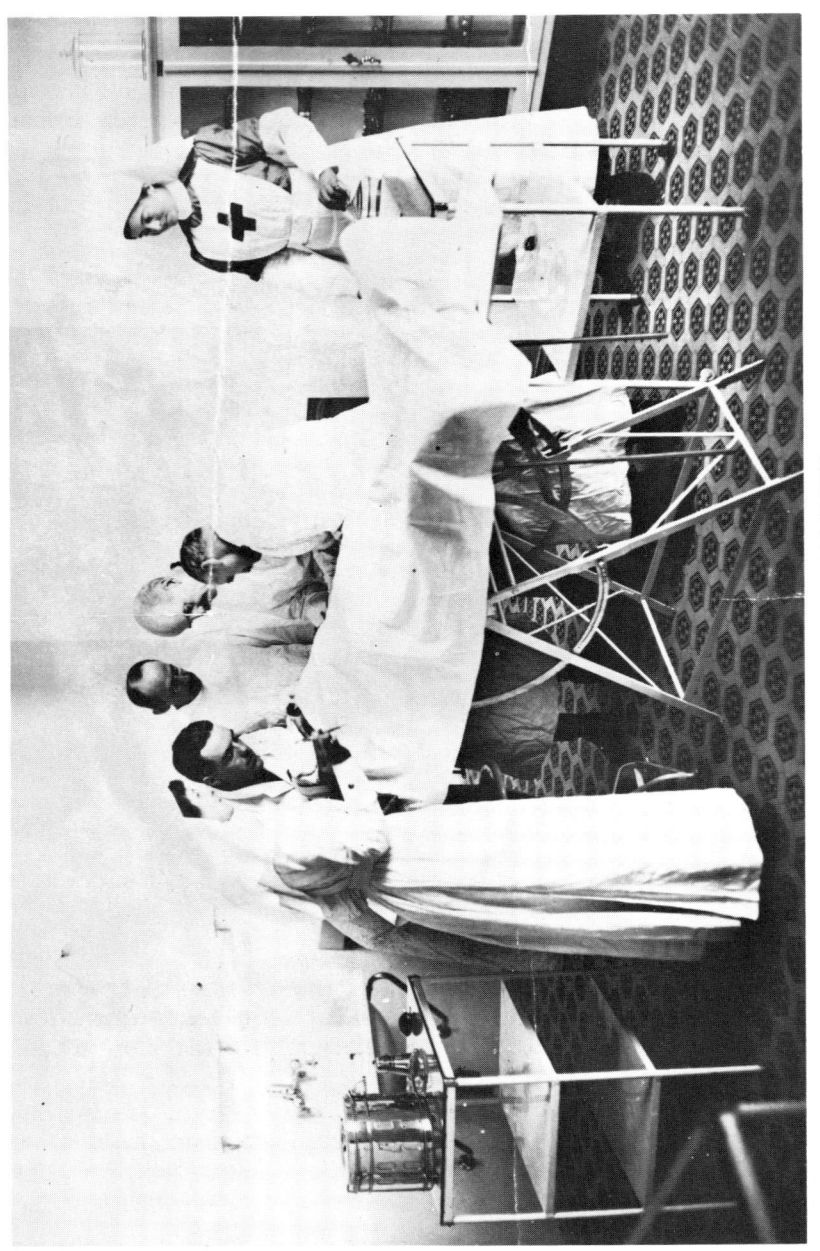

OPERATING IN THE HOSPITAL

in the hospital at that time and to her husband she wrote: 'Had one v. anxious case of amputation of the arm (gas-gangrene). He is living still although Harmer said he could not live more than 2 days'. Nor is even that the end of the story; for Blunt in his biography records that in 1931 Lady Muriel came across this same Russian officer selling newspapers on the streets of Paris.

A somewhat startling suggestion relating to this disease may also be mentioned. A previous chapter told something of the effects of the newly developed technique of aerial bombardment, a mere token of course of what was to be experienced in later wars. One of these effects provoked the following comment from the authors of the *BMJ* article:

> One of us, prior to visiting Russia, had a terrible experience of the wounds caused by bombs dropped from Zeppelins, as he had been surgeon for the day at Charing Cross Hospital when the Zeppelin raid took place in September 1915. On this occasion 100 patients were admitted into Charing Cross Hospital, of whom fourteen were dead on admission, and nine others died within twelve hours. In every wound examined bacteriologically the *Bacillus aerogenes capsulatus* was identified. The same organism was found in every case of wound caused by a bomb dropped from an aeroplane admitted into the Petrograd hospital. The fact that in every Zeppelin and aeroplane bomb wound examined at Charing Cross Hospital and the Petrograd hospital the *B. aerogenes capsulatus* was demonstrated, makes us suspect that the outer casing of the bomb must have been infected with a culture of this micro-organism. If such be the case, science has surely never before been made to serve so fiendish a purpose.

This was surely coincidental. I do not doubt the integrity of the writers, nor do I think that this was 'propaganda' since I have never come across another such account. It is now well recognised that all urban and rural detritus is contaminated with the spores of tetanus and gas-gangrene bacilli, which exist quite happily in the intestines of humans and other animals, particularly horses of which there were still many in the streets of London in 1915. Moreover, when a bullet or a piece of shrapnel, travelling at high velocity, enters human tissue it sucks-in the clothing of the victim, itself contaminated. Nonetheless this makes one recall the assertion by the 'Red Dean', Dr. Hewlett Johnston, who stated as a fact when he visited Peking during the

Chinese Civil War in 1950, that the Americans were spraying plague bacilli from the air.

On a lighter note one may mention an account given by Jefferson of the attempt to instruct the physician Gould May into the intricacies of surgery: 'To-day May did three minor operations with Waterhouse acting as his 'dresser'. It was a perfect pantomime! I also extracted my first bullet from a patient to-day and was naturally very pleased. Unfortunately all the trophies have to go to the patients . . .' He gave a more chilling description of the first occasion on which he had to remove an eye and although he described with explicit detail this harrowing operation I would wish to spare the reader such details.

Two other common medical problems are also worth a record: the first bizarre, the second surprising. The incidence of roundworm infestation amongst Russian soldiers at that time was astonishingly high. This did not seem to worry the 'host' but, for the anaesthetist who was inducing a patient for operation, the sudden appearance of a number of worms in the mask was anything but reassuring. WDH himself, opening an abdomen to suture a ruptured intestine, confessed himself shaken to find three *Ascaris lumbricoides* milling about in the general mess inside the peritoneal cavity! Trench foot, which is actually a form of frostbite-gangrene, was one of the most incapacitating conditions resulting from the mud and cold of the trenches on the Western Front during the winter months. Surprisingly it seems rarely to have occurred on the Eastern Front. 'To our astonishment, we saw far fewer cases than we encountered in the various London hospitals. The Russian soldier knows nothing about socks or stockings. He wraps his foot in a square piece of flannel and then puts on an excellent loose-fitting top boot. Despite the fact that he has to face a temperature 30° to 40° lower than that encountered by his British comrade, he is far less liable to suffer from frostbite or trench feet. Admittedly he is more inured to extremes of cold, but as the result of our experiences we recommend, as the best way to prevent frostbite and trench feet, a flannel wrap around the foot and a loosely-fitting top-boot.'

The *BMJ* article makes no mention of poison gas though patients suffering from its effects must surely have passed through their wards. The Germans had used this new and devastating weapon on the Eastern Front as early as June 1915, though their first major attack was launched on the night of 6th July. Scotland Liddell records that the gas-shells on the Bzura-Rawka Front killed or disabled 3300 men during this one attack. 'Yet each man had a respirator and goggles to protect them from the searing acid and the officers were confident of their effectiveness. "Then why?" I asked an Officer. He shrugged his shoulders. "Russia's a queer country", he said, "there are things you will never understand. The men were not ordered to put them on". I was inclined to doubt his word but some days later I mentioned the matter to some officers of higher rank. "But that could never be?" I said. "It's possible", said they.'

There were other pests which decimated the forces as well. On the Southern Fronts the *Anopheles* mosquito occurred in myriad numbers and malaria was universal. 'The highly-polluted water is largely drunk unboiled (complained a BRCS Report) and briefly, military hygiene, as understood in the West, is almost unknown, or unpractised, on this Front . . .' Further north, in the Pripet Marshes, were the flies: flies in such fantastic numbers that writers ran out of hyperbole in attempting to describe them. The narrator of *The Dark Forest* did his best. 'Then there are the Flies. I write them with a capital letter because I've got to keep my head above the Flies. Does anyone at home or away from this infernal strip of fighting realise what flies are? Of course one's read of the tropical sort . . . what you like, evil and horrid, but these here are just the ordinary household kind. Quite ordinary, but sheets, *walls* of them. I came into our little larder this morning. I thought they'd painted the place black during the night. Then, at my taking the cover off some sugar, it was exactly as if the walls hovered and fell inward.'

And in their train of course followed infection, corruption and disease. Above all they were necrophyllic.

The dead were buried each evening in communal pits; 'fraternal graves' they were called, since Russian, German, Austrian and Polish soldiers — civilians too — were interred regardless of their nationality. 'There they lay at peace in a brothers' grave', wrote *Krestovaya Sestra* Florence Farmborough after she had visited one such grave at dusk to scatter flowers within it. 'Swarms of flies added to the horror and covered the dead brothers as with a thick black pall. I remember the feeling of horror when I first saw what I had imagined to be a layer of earth and then that the whole black pall was *moving*.'

During the latter half of 1917 the base hospital in Petrograd was given over largely to medical cases and among these were a number suffering from scurvy, a disease caused by a deficiency of vitamin C. A report to the London Committee mentions that Dr Rosher was preparing 'A Study of Fifty Cases of Scurvy' but I am not able to find evidence of its publication.

143

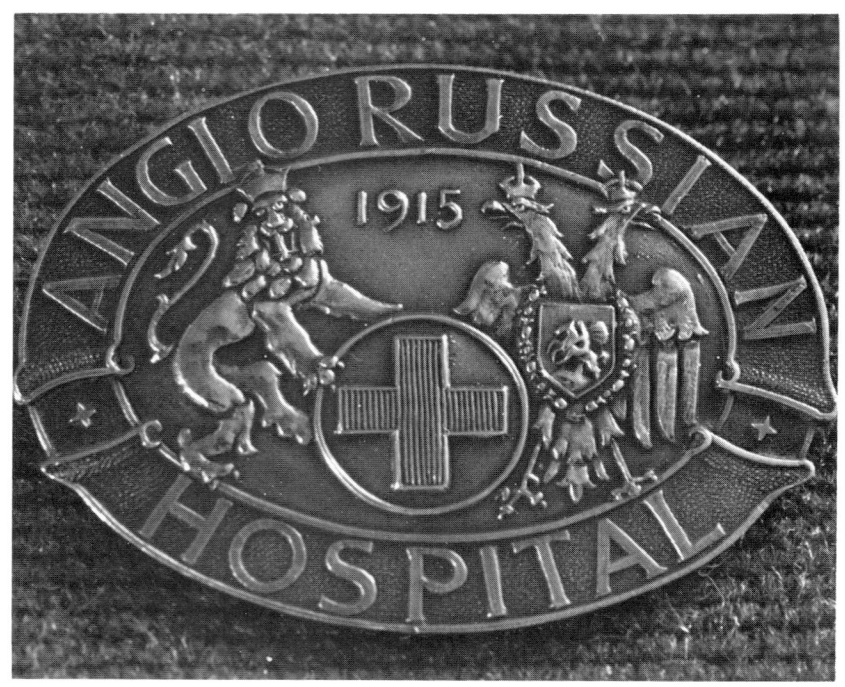

THE BADGE OF THE HOSPITAL

One is bound to admit that very little practical information came from the medical staff of the hospital. Consequently, although this chapter ought to provide the evidence in justification for the work of the A-R H., it is difficult to do so. The questions have to be asked: Was the effort of the London Committee and the involvement of the British Red Cross Society rewarded? Did the subscribers get their money's worth? How much did it really aid the Russian allies? I do not think these questions are capable of answer: at any rate I do not believe that I can answer them. But at least I can place some financial evidence before the reader.

In November 1917 the London Committee published a Report about the work of the Hospital.[4] An Introductory Note by Lord

[4] *The Work of the Anglo-Russian Hospital: September 1915 to June 1917.* Andrew M. Fleming CMG, MBCM, FRCS, DPH and Geoffrey Jefferson MS, FRCS. This report is of much importance insofar as it has provided many details which I have been able to include in previous chapters.

Cheylesmore began by recording with sadness the deaths of the President of the Fund, Lord Cromer and of the Vice-Chairman of his own Executive Committee, Sir Starr Jameson. The bulk of it consisted of a simple and factual account of the medical and surgical activities of the several hospitals which had operated between the winter of 1915 and the summer of 1917. But it was really a kind of Annual Report to the shareholders of a Company because it also included a Balance Sheet — 'A Statement of the Receipts and Payments in London and Petrograd': and from this one may observe some interesting figures. A total of £107,480 1s. 1d. had been received in subscriptions, donations and interest. Outgoings had amounted to £61,824 6s. 6d., leaving a healthy balance of £45,655 14s. 7d. A mere £2,300 had been spent on Administration and Staff Salaries and wages accounted for just over £10,000. Even the motor column, which was in some ways the pride of the organisation, only cost £486 10s. 5d. It may be protested that such figures are meaningless. They are not! Let anyone refer to Appendix 3 and calculate, if he will, the salaries in to-day's terms of 22 doctors,[5] 62 nurses, four orderlies, 19 chauffeurs and two secretaries.

The finances are certainly complicated by the fact that the BRCS also contributed to the running expenses, commencing to do so in September 1916 and assuming full responsibility after July 1917. So, to the outgoings of roughly £62,000 incurred by the A-R H. itself and which covered the whole of its first year's work and a part of its second, there must be added the sum of £109,572 which the BRCS spent between September 1916 and the closure of the Hospital. One can at least say with certainty that the subscribers got their money's worth.

Statistically it is true that about 6,000 patients were treated and that the mortality was less than one per cent in the base hospital in Petrograd and between four and five per cent in the field hospitals. As the Russians learned to trust the British surgeons they sent them more severe casualties and so the mortality rose. Over 50 per cent of deaths were due to gas-gangrene. There was of course no follow-up. Casualties were seldom kept in the field hospitals for more than a week: if they had not died, they were evacuated. By agreement with the Russian authorities those in Petrograd had to be kept until they could

---

[5] In 1980 a newly qualified hospital doctor received £5,400 p.a. — plus increments. As a house-surgeon at Bart's in 1938 I was paid £20 p.a. — plus my laundry. In one of his letters to his wife, Jefferson remarks with some satisfaction that 'my rate of pay has just been put up to 24/- per day, i.e. £436 per annum'.

be discharged, either back to their units or to wherever they had come from in that immense land. This itself limited the turn-over of beds to a great extent. Since it seems impossible for me to make a genuine assessment, I will let Dr Andrew Fleming write for me; brave words perhaps, but not empty words:

> We had established a Base Hospital in the Capital second to none; we had organised in the field two most useful units, and had running a large fleet of motor ambulances, which was of immense value at the Russian front with its great distances and absence of railway facilities. We had, moreover, established good relations with our Russian allies, and had been to them a sign manual of British appreciation and sympathy.

Epilogue

I began this Essay saying that it had a hero and two heroines and that, of the latter, I thought Lady Sybil had won by a short head. In completing it I am not so sure. It was a photo-finish certainly and I must leave the judgment to my readers. In any case it seems proper that I should end with some sort of summing up of my main *dramatis personae.*

Lady Sybil, unquestionably, was perfect for the job she took over in November 1915. She was actually in Russia longer than Lady Muriel and but for her unlucky injury and the terminal illness of her father in 1917, I doubt if she would have returned to England at all while the hospital was in being. She wrote trenchantly of what she considered the failings of her subordinates — even offensively on occasion — but she did so in the sure conviction that her upbringing entitled her to do so. To-day I suppose that would be called arrogance: in those days it was acceptable and in my view it was right. Filial piety requires that I should record that in all the letters which I have read and which passed between Lady Muriel and Lady Sybil, my father seems to have been almost the only member of the medical staff who escaped, for one reason or another, the lash of their pens! Though she did not return to Russia, she went out to France, succeeding Lady Loch as Overseas Commandant of the Womens' Legion RASC and there she remained until she retired from this post in April 1920. Her OBE was awarded her in 1918 and so one may assume that this was for her work with the Anglo-Russian Hospital.

Her son Harry Middleton tells me that his mother loved talking about her experiences and in this respect she seems to have differed from all the rest of those who I have attempted to portray. As a BBC man himself he naturally regrets the absence of 'tape' in those days, for although Lady Sybil often considered committing herself in print she never succeeded in doing so. She kept up her interest in the British Red Cross Society between the wars and during World War Two played a prominent part in the organisation of the Scottish branches of the Red Cross. Her enthusiasm and her warm heart pervades these pages.

Lady Muriel's life was well documented by Wilfrid Blunt in 1962 as I have often indicated. But from what I have learned myself it may be possible to add a little or even to correct in some degree the impression which he gives of her personality. Her family have suggested that Blunt over-emphasised her waywardness, perhaps confusing her with her mother, Lady Winchilsea, who even by Victorian standards was quite unusually eccentric. She was I am assured rather conventional: 'There was nothing weird or exotic about her, though her mind was undisciplined and unbusinesslike'. Thus Pamela Glenconner, who added the delightful suggestion that Blunt's biography should really have been called 'Six Impossible Things Before Breakfast', which she generally set out to do and which, as is well known, the Red Queen in *Through the Looking Glass* accomplished each day. She had a quiet voice, a persuasive manner and a keen sense of humour. She was in a constant rush, enjoyed publicity and fund-raising and her two secretaries never had time to do anything but the most urgent work before something else equally important turned up. She made friends with the greatest of ease in all classes of society, yet never doubted her own heritage.

Tamara Talbot-Rice, who has helped me in Russian matters, recalls how she met Lady Muriel in Leningrad in 1935 when she attended the first Art Congress held by the Soviets. 'These were dangerous times (she wrote to me) and my mother was distressed at my going. Christopher Sykes and Robert Byron were also attending and had elected to stay with Muriel. This led to hideous complications. I met Muriel and we instantly took to each other. She made me confess my plans and instantly forbade them as too dangerous to those involved. The great purge amongst those who had been in contact with foreigners followed several months later and proved her to have been right. My affection and admiration of her steadily increased; so did my admiration for Sir Richard, whom she really shelved in order to run her Home [for Distressed British Subjects] in Russia.'

On an occasion when Lady Muriel was coming round after an anaesthetic, a nurse said to her: 'Everything is quite all right Lady Paget'; to which she answered firmly: 'I am not *Lady Paget!*' Some of her many illnesses were surely self-induced and if she was a victim of psychoneurosis, the definition 'a conflict between a wish and its fulfilment', has at least a charitable sound. Her motto was *Never Say Die* and in truth she carried this to the end. The fact that she was treated with 'deep X-rays' by the great Doctor Couthard in Paris and consulted Sir Lenthal Cheatle in London provides a clear diagnosis for any surgeon: and this is confirmed by a remark which she made to a friend that she 'felt she was falling apart' — the classical description of those suffering from osteolytic metastases. A harassed young official at the Foreign Office, Mr Jack Greenaway, once wrote a delightful little piece of doggerel about her:

How lucky Lady Muriel
isn't in the pluriel!

and I think that this may perhaps serve as the nicest of epitaphs. It is indeed impossible not to speculate on what she might have accomplished in the Second World War had she been spared in 1938.

My father was a modest man. When Lady Sybil wrote that he was 'rather weak but I think his other qualities outweigh this', I know very well what she meant. Sixty-four years later Pamela Glenconner was able to tell me that 'your father was well-liked. He was clearly a brave, sensible, well-qualified man who gave up a good practice to go on this small scale adventurous expedition to help the Russian allies. He must have been a tower of strength and did splendid work. He had a great respect for Lady Sybil but less patience with the "monstrous regiment of women" in general and their unreliable amateur ways'. As I have recounted, my father never really enjoyed good health and looking back it must seem pretty crazy that, so soon after his severe attack of tuberculosis, he submitted himself to the Russian climate and that in time of war. Later, he suffered from severe allergic conditions and a duodenal ulcer, for which he was operated upon at the age of 79. The death of my mother from acute pancreatitis, when they were on holiday together in New Zealand, was a devastating event, yet he lived into his ninetieth year. In his own field of surgery he was supreme, being in particular a pioneer in the treatment of cancer of the larynx by radium, a method which obviated the necessity of removing the larynx and thereby leaving the patient more or less speechless.

My father kept up his association with the A-R H. and saw many of its personnel in subsequent years. Lady Sybil remained most generous in her affection — 'I wish you could see my face: it is wonderful, *thanks to you!*': and I remember meeting both her and Lady Muriel in our own home when I was a boy. Had WDH returned to Russia in 1917, as they wished him to do, he would no doubt have presided over the demise of the hospital and perhaps this would have led to a more lasting friendship. Who can say?

149

I wish to express to you & to all the Doctors & Surgeons who worked in the Auxiliary Hospitals during the Great War, my deep appreciation of your splendid Services. I feel unable to thank you personally, as I should wish to do - & I therefore ask you to accept with the accompanying War Medal of the "British Red Cross" Society, my warmest & most grateful thanks for the Services you rendered with such generous unselfish devotion to the Sick & wounded under your Care!

Alexandra

May 1921 -

H.M. QUEEN ALEXANDRA'S LETTER

The Anglo-Russian Hospital was the Empire's gift to Russia. 'In this form', the original Appeal of 1915 stated, 'we give a practical sign of our deep and growing admiration and gratitude toward those who throughout the Russian Empire are fighting so valiantly against the common enemy. As a National Gift the Hospital is being received in Russia. It has the active support of the British Government. Every part of our Empire is joining in the tribute'.

This was the 'gesture' which His Majesty's Ambassador, Sir George Buchanan had advised the Foreign Office would be appreciated by the Russians in 1915. The offer was indeed welcomed by the Empress Marie who, as Head of the Russian Red Cross had replied by telegram:

> *May I ask you to express my warmest gratitude to the Committee for the beautiful gift, and for their kind offer of further assistance to the Russian Red Cross Society.*

The gift survived for little more than two years and a feeling of disappointment, an aura of failure even, remains in the mind of the biographer. Had I been asked to review this Essay myself, I think I would have written (though I would have done so in the most compassionate terms) that its author had made the best of a bad job. It was not the fault of the A-R H. Committee and most certainly not that of my two heroines. The simple fact is that the hospital was in the wrong place and this accounts for the endless discussions amongst the medical staff as to what could be done about it and it also explains why Lady Muriel was always rushing off to the Front in order to try and find something better.

Herein lay the paradox. The roots of the Anglo-Russian Hospital lay in St Petersburg and I use the old name of the city deliberately because this was where the Royal family, the Embassy and the Foreign Office were able to exert their influence. Without the 'establishment' the hospital would have withered, for Moscow had barely enough facilities and were scarcely interested in having the British to complicate their own serious problems. Kiev was where the A-R H. should have been, as the young Jefferson observed and indeed where Lady Muriel persistently tried to locate it. She failed as I have shown because there was an insufficient liaison between Petrograd and the army commanders in the battle-zone of the South-Western Front.

The hopes and expectations of those who nurtured the hospital may not have been fully realised but none can doubt the enthusiasm and integrity of those who begat it: and who shall compute the number of lives saved, the suffering alleviated in the living and dying by such a small band of immensely skilled, dedicated and most courageous women and men?

Six years later my father received a letter.

> *Marlborough House*
>
> *I wish to express to you and to all the Doctors & Surgeons who worked in the Domiciliary Hospital during the Great War my deep appreciation of your splendid Services. I am unable to thank you personally as I should wish to do & I therefore ask you to accept with the accompanying War Medal of the 'British Red Cross Society', my warmest & most grateful thanks for the Services you rendered with such generous unselfish devotion to the Sick & wounded under your care!*
>
> *May 1921*   Alexandra

The Dowager Queen Mother was 71 years of age when she wrote this, in her own firm hand, on black-edged paper bearing her cypher and in the blackest of inks, although King Edward VII had been dead for more than 11 years. The Queen herself died four years later and with the death of its Patroness this was the end of the Anglo-Russian Hospital.

Apart from the splendid Icon and the documents in the British Red Cross Society's archives, what else remains of *The Forgotten Hospital?* Many letters, a small diary, a few photographs and a bronze Uniform Badge. And memories of course; the memories of those few who knew and admired the people who took part in this enterprise.

When I myself was in Leningrad in 1965 I stood before the Dmitri Palace. It was then a Government Office— Number 41 Nevsky Prospekt. In 1926 when Lady Muriel Paget re-visited it for the last time she found that it had become a People's Club. It is fitting that her own words should conclude my Essay.

> In the little Chapel behind the Great Staircase the altar had disappeared. In place of the 'unprogressive' *lampada* and ikon there was an electrically-lit photograph of Lenin.

Appendices

Chronology of the Anglo-Russian Hospital

All dates are given in terms of the Western calendar which was 13 days 'in advance' of the Russian calendar.

1915

August	Establishment of the London Committee under the Patronage of HM Queen Alexandra, with the Earl of Cromer as President, Major-General Lord Cheylesmore as Chairman of the Executive Committee and Lady Muriel Paget as Honorary Organising Secretary.
	Issue of Prospectuses and Appeal.
	Engagement of Medical, Nursing and Ancillary Staff.
October (mid)	Advance party left from Newcastle, via Norway, Sweden and Finland, to Petrograd: Lady Sybil Grey (*vice* Lady Muriel Paget), Mr Ian Malcolm MP, Dr Fleming (Commandant) and the Grand Duchess, 'Countess' Olga.
October 24	The Dmitri Palace offered as Base Hospital.
October 30	Main party left from London to Archangel: Miss Irvine Robertson (Matron), nurses and VADs, junior medical staff.
November 24	Senior staff left from Newcastle via Norway, Sweden and Finland to Petrograd: Messrs Waterhouse and Harmer, Doctors Gould May and Flavelle, Miss Bates (Assistant Matron).
Nov. to Dec.	Conversion of Dmitri Palace. An exceptionally cold winter.

1916

January 25	Presentation of Icon to the A-R H. Committee.
February 1	Official opening of the hospital by the Grand Duchess Vladimir.

April 25	Arrival of Lady Muriel Paget in Petrograd.
June 4	Brusilov Offensive opened at Lutsk, south of the Pripet Marshes.
June 7	Blessing of the Field Hospital at the Corps des Pages and its departure for Volhynia four days later.
June 18	Lady Sybil Grey injured at Voropayevo and her subsequent return to England.
July 23	Field Hospital moved to Rovno and Lutsk.
July 28-30	Battle of the River Stokhod.
July	A-R H. Fund raising matinée in London.
August 31	Dr Fleming returned to England.
October (mid)	Lady Sybil Grey returned to Russia.
October	Field Hospital moved to the Bukovina and the Motor Column established.
October 15	Mr Waterhouse returned to England.
October 23	Mr Harmer returned to England.
November 1	Dr Flavelle took up post of Commandant. Lady Muriel Paget returned to England.
Oct. to Dec.	Field Hospital and Motor Column active on the Carpathian Front.
November (mid)	Battle of Kirli-Baba.
December 29	Rasputin assassinated.
	1917
January 20	The Matron, Miss Irvine Robertson, returned to England.
Jan. to Feb.	Increasing administrative difficulties in Petrograd.
March 8	Uprising in Petrograd.
March 14	Issue of Army Order Number One.
March 15	Abdication of Tsar Nicholas II.
April 16	Arrival of Lenin and other Bolshevik leaders in Petrograd.
May	A-R H. Exhibition in London.
End of May	Lady Muriel Paget returned to Russia.
June 29	Russian offensive opened against the Austro-German forces in the Carpathians.
July 16	Bolshevik rising in Petrograd.
End of July	Lady Sybil Grey returned to England.
August	Lady Muriel Paget contracted typhoid fever.
November 6	The Bolshevik Revolution.
December 17	Armistice between Russia and the Central Powers.

ACTIVE SERVICE OF THE STAFF OF THE HOSPITAL

	1915	1916	1917	1918
Lady Muriel Paget				
Lady Sybil Grey				
Dr Andrew Fleming				
Mr Herbert Waterhouse				
Mr Douglas Harmer				
Dr John Flavelle				
Dr Gould May				
Miss Irvine Robertson				
Dr H. F. Q. Thompson				
Mr Geoffrey Jefferson				
Mr Jennings Marshall				
Dr Walter Yeld				

HOSPITAL OPENED

HOSPITAL CLOSED

1918

January 18	Closure of Base Hospital in Petrograd and evacuation through Finland.
End of February	Lady Muriel Paget left Kiev with the Field Hospital for Odessa.
March 3	Treaty of Brest Litovsk.
March 7	Lady Muriel Paget took the remaining British personnel from Moscow, via Siberia, Japan and the USA, to England.
May 26	Arrival at Liverpool.
July 16	Murder of the Tsar and his family at Ekaterinburg.

1921

Presentation of the Icon to the British Red Cross Society by Lady Sybil Middleton.

1925

November 20	Death of HM Queen Alexandra, Patroness of the Hospital.

Appendix 2

The Committee of The Anglo-Russian Hospital

Patroness
HER MAJESTY QUEEN ALEXANDRA

President
The Rt. Hon. The Earl of Cromer, PC, GCB, etc.

Vice-Presidents

The Most Reverend The Archbishop of Canterbury

The Most Reverend The Archbishop of York	The Rt. Hon. The Lord Mayor of London
The Rt. Hon. H. H. Asquith	Admiral Lord Charles Beresford, GCB
The Rt. Hon. Arthur J. Balfour	The Rt. Hon. Lord Farquhar
Field Mar. Earl Kitchener, KP	Field Mar. The Rt. Hon. Lord Grenfell, GCB
The Rt. Hon. Sir Edward Grey, Bart, KG	Lord Weardale
The Rt. Hon. Earl Curzon of Kedleston	Lord Sydenham of Combe, GCSI
The Rt. Hon. Walter H. Long	The Rt. Hon. Sir William Mather
The Rt. Hon. Austen Chamberlain	General The Rt. Hon. Sir Arthur Paget
The Rt. Hon. A. Bonar Law	Sir Donald Mackenzie Wallace, KCVO

157

General Committee

The Lord Provost of Aberdeen
Mr Herbert Allen
Rt. Hon. Lord Ampthill
Sir Kenneth S. Anderson, KCMG
Mr H. T. Baker
Lord Balfour of Burleigh
Mr Archibald Balfour
The Bishop of Bangor
Hon. Maurice Baring
Mr H. W. Barnett
Sir Edward Beauchamp, Bart, MP
Miss Benenson
Lieut.-Gen. Sir E. C. Bethune, KCB, CVO
Mr W. J. Birkbeck
Rt. Hon. The Lord Mayor of Birmingham
Sir Samuel B. Boulton, Bart
Rt. Hon. Earl Brassey, GCB
Mr J. A. Bryce, MP
Hon. Edward Cadogan
Lord Hugh Cecil, MP
Sir Valentine Chirol
Mr Stanley Christopherson
Sir James B. Dale, Bart
Mr Geoffrey Drage
The Lord Provost of Edinburgh
Baron Emile Erlanger
Sir Edward Evans
Bishop of Exeter
Sir Algernon F. Firth, Bart
Mr Seymour Fort
Mr T. B. Gabriel
Mr J. Gallatly
Hon. Herbert Gibbs
The Worshipful The Mayor of Grimsby

Lady Hanbury Williams
Mr G. Booth Heming
Mr J. J. Hughes
Sir John Jackson, MP
Rt. Hon. The Lord Mayor of Leeds
Mr C. F. H. Leslie
Mrs Lessing
Mr G. A. Lloyd, MP
Hon. Francis McLaren, MP
Rt. Hon. The Lord Mayor of Manchester
Mr S. F. Mendl
Rt. Hon. Lord Nunburnholme
Rt. Hon. Sir Arthur Nicholson, GCB
Bishop of Ossory
Professor Bernard Pares
Rt. Hon. Lord Parmoor, KCVO
Viscount Peel
Sir William Plender
Rt. Hon. Lord Ribblesdale
The Marchioness of Ripon
Lord Sanderson
Mr A. Serena, JP
Rt. Hon. Lord Southwark
Rt. Hon. Sir Albert Spicer, MP
Hon. Arthur Stanley, CVO, MP
Mr J. Herbert Tritton
Sir William Vestey, Bart
Bishop of Wakefield
The Rt. Worship. The Mayor of Westminster
Mr Richard White
Lieut.-Gen. Sir J. Wolfe Murray, KCB
Mr C. T. Hagberg Wright
Col. Charles E. Yate, MP

Executive Committee

Chairman: Major-General Lord Cheylesmore, KCVO
Vice-Chairman: The Rt. Hon. Sir Starr Jameson, Bart
Hon. Treasurer: Sir Owen Philipps, KCMG
Hon. Organising Secretary: Lady Muriel Paget
Hon. Secretary: Mr Oliver Williams

The Hon. Evelyn Hubbard
Sir William Mather, PC
Mr Harry Cust
Mr F. S. Clarke
Mr Herbert Guedalla
Mr John Buchan
Mr Richard Burbridge
Mr Ian Malcolm, MP

Lady Cheylesmore
Lady (Arthur) Paget
Lady Juliet Duff
The Hon. Mrs Jasper Ridley
Lady Egerton
Lady Philipps
Mrs Walter Long
Mrs H. F. Wood

158

List of Members of Staff of the Anglo-Russian Hospital

(This document was found among Lady Muriel Paget's papers and was probably compiled about November 1917.)

Medical Staff

Dr Andrew M. Fleming
Sir H. F. Waterhouse
Dr William Lingard
Mr W. Douglas Harmer
Dr Aron Pastel
Dr C. Gould May
Capt W. B. Macdermott
Dr Edward Rivera
Dr Mark Gardner
Major J. G. Hunt
Dr H. Q. F. Thompson

Dr W. H. Yeld
Dr J. M. Flavelle
Dr Graham Aspland
Dr G. A. Jones
Mr Geoffrey Jefferson
Dr A. B. Rosher
Dr A. H. Sevier
Dr Sydney Williams
Mr C. J. Marshall
Mr G. C. Bott
Mr H. Harrison

Nursing Staff and VAD's

Miss S. S. Irvine Robertson
Miss Dorothy Bates
Miss Alice Adcock
Miss Alice Bateman
Miss Emily Boykett
Miss Beatrice Carlill
Miss Dorothy Cotton
Miss Hannah Hancock
Miss Lucy Hayes
Miss Florence Ingram
Miss Helen Macdonald
Miss Kelly
Miss Mary MacDonald
Miss Jessie Mavor
Miss Dorothy Nicholls
Miss Albina Pinniger
Miss Mary Ann Price
Miss Winifred Sturt
Miss Jessie Sutherland
Miss Gertrude Squire
Miss Ada Maria Webb
Miss Elizabeth Jones
Miss G. O. Hopkins
Miss Ann Scrymgeour-Wedderburn
Miss Hettie Whitehouse
Miss Emily Thomson
Miss Effie Turner
Miss Evelina Alexander

Miss Martha Davies
Miss H. Davies
Miss Marguerite Farrow
Miss Elizabeth Farrow
Miss Christine Hunter
Miss Margaret Gorrie
Miss Edith Hegan
Miss Eleanor Chance
Miss E. Marion Dawson
Miss Florence M. McLeod
Miss Ethel B. Lyall
Miss Mildred Mitchener
Miss McCallum
Miss Ena Stevenson
Miss Gladys A. D. Statter
Miss Florence White Tait
Miss Enid Stocker
Miss Isabella Grant
Miss Cicely Buchan
Miss Judkins
Miss Bird
Miss I. B. Welsh
Miss M. K. Lloyd
Miss Curtis
Miss Holloway
Miss Angus
Miss B. Agnes Conway
Miss Maclennan

	Miss Florence Barrington	Miss Strange
	Miss Hilda Bewicke	Miss Cooke
	Miss Mary M. Carter	
Orderlies	Mr Frances MacNally	Mr John Whittingdale
	Mr Lyndall Pocock	Mr Bingham
Chauffeurs	Mr Samuel Wyatt	Mr A. E. Dickinson
	Mr Digby Jones	Mr P. Hart
	Mr Mills	Mr P. Keeble
	Mr William Compton	Mr W. W. D. Bryden
	Mr Dixon	Mr R. F. Parsons
	Mr Arthur Turner	Mr H. R. Wright
	Mr Harold Robinson	Mr J. H. King
	Mr W. Lyon Blease	Mr L. F. Torkington
	Mr W. D. Tysson	Mr A. H. Mander
	Mr James Norman (Deceased)	
Secretaries	Miss Janet Crawford	Miss Hilda Jameson

The Russian Royal Family

who were associated with the Hospital.

The Tsarina. Princess Alexandra (Alix) of Hesse-Darmstadt, *alias* Alexandra Federovna, wife of Tsar Nicholas II.

The Dowager Empress. Princess Dagmar of Denmark, *alias* Marie Federovna, widow of Tsar Alexander III and sister of Queen Alexandra, widow of King Edward VII of Great Britain. Patroness of the Hospital.

The Grand Duchess Vladimir. Princess Marie (Meichen) of Mecklenburg-Schwerein, *alias* Marie Pavlovna; widow of the Grand Duke Vladimir, eldest brother of Tsar Alexander III.

The Grand Duke Sergius. Younger brother of the Grand Duke Vladimir; married the Tsarina's eldest sister Elizabeth (Ella) and was murdered while serving as Governor-General of Moscow in 1914.

The Grand Duchess Serge. Widow of the Grand Duke Sergius. She became Abbess of the Miséricorde Convent following her husband's death and ran a medical service, of which it is said that the Grand Duchess Vladimir was jealous. Owner of the Dmitri Palace, which she gave to her nephew:—

The Grand Duke Dmitri, who was therefore a nephew by marriage of the Tsar. His cousin Irine married:—

Prince Feliks Yusoupov, who was therefore a relation by marriage of Dmitri and in whose Palace on the Moika Rasputin was murdered.

The Grand Duke Cyril. Son of the Grand Duke Vladimir and who, after the murder of the Tsar and his family, became the head of the Romanov dynasty. Following his death his son, Vladimir (born 1917), became the claimant.

The Russian Red Cross

Officials associated with the Hospital.

PETROGRAD
Mr Polutsov (one of the five Heads of the RRC)
Colonel Alexander Fénoult, a member of the Imperial Guard (Lady Sybil's 'personal slave')
General Leman (Commandant of Dmitri Hospital)

THE FIELD
Mr Boris Ignatiev
Baron Meyendorf
Mr Martens
Mr Alexis Homiakov
Advisers to the Hospital
Professor Willheminov
RRC District Commandant

Notes on the Illustrations

Page 7

WILLIAM DOUGLAS HARMER, MC(Cantab), FRCS(Eng)
1873-1962. Portrait by Edmund Brock, ARA 1913 when he
was 40 years of age.

Page 13

LADY MURIEL PAGET, CBE. A photograph taken in 1922 in
Prague. She wears a uniform designed by herself for the 'Paget
Mission' to Slovakia. Provided by Pamela Lady Glenconner her
daughter.

Page 21

LADY SYBIL GREY, OBE. A photograph taken in 1920. She wears
the uniform of the Womens' Legion RASC. Provided by
Mr Harry Middleton her son.

Page 42

THE HOSPITAL STAFF. A photograph taken about April 1916. In
the front row (left to right and amongst others) are WDH,
Lady Sybil Grey, the Matron, Lady Muriel Paget and Dr
Andrew Fleming. In the second row are Dr Mark Gardner, the
Assistant Matron Miss Bates and Dr Gould May.

Page 51

THE GREAT STAIRCASE, with staff and patients. A BRCS
photograph. In the centre are the Matron Miss Irvine Robertson, Dr Fleming and Lady Sybil Grey; behind the last is
WDH.

Page 59

THE DMITRI PALACE. In the original photograph of the Palace
the lettering on the board over the main entrance, which
proclaims the name of the hospital, can just be decyphered. One
of the four bronze horses, which stand at each corner of the
Fontanka Bridge, may also be identified. A BRCS photograph.

Sources and References

BOOKS

ALEXINSKY, T. *With the Russian Wounded,* 1916. Ministry of Defence Library (Central & Army).

BEGBIE, Harold. *Albert, Fourth Earl Grey:* A Last Word. (Hodder & Stoughton, 1918).

BLUNT, Wilfrid. *Lady Muriel:* Lady Muriel Paget, her Husband and her Philanthropic Work in Central and Eastern Europe. (Methuen & Co., 1962).

THE BRITISH RED CROSS SOCIETY. *Joint War Committee Reports, 1914-1919.*

BUCHANAN, Meriel. *Victorian Gallery.* (Cassell, 1956).

COWLES, Virginia. *The Last Tsar and Tsarina.* (Weidenfield and Nicolson, 1978.)

FARMBOROUGH, Florence, FRGS. *Nurse at the Russian Front:* A Diary 1914-1918. (Constable, 1974).

KNOX, Major-General Sir A. *With the Russian Army,* 1914-1917. Extracts from the diary of a military attaché. Ministry of Defence Library (Central & Army).

KRIPPNER, Monica. *The Quality of Mercy.* (David & Charles, 1980).

LIDDELL, R. Scotland. *On the Russian Front.* (Simpkin, Marshall, Hamilton & Kent, 1916).

MASSIE, Robert. *Nicholas and Alexandra.* (Gollancz, 1968).

McLAREN, Barbara. *Women of the War.* (Hodder & Stoughton, 1917).

MITCHELL, David. *Women on the Warpath:* The Story of Women in the First World War. (Jonathan Cape, 1966).

OLIVER, Beryl, GBE, RRC. *The British Red Cross in Action.* (Faber & Faber, 1966).

PARES, Bernard, KBE. *My Russian Memoirs.* (Jonathan Cape, 1931).

THE ROYAL COLLEGE OF SURGEONS OF ENGLAND. *Lives of the Fellows.* (1953).

STOPFORD, The Hon. Albert. [Published anonymously]. *The Russian Diary Of An Englishman.* (William Heinemann, 1919).

WALPOLE, Hugh. *The Dark Forest.* (Macmillan, 1916).

YOUSOUPOFF, Prince. *Rasputin.* [English translation by Oswald Rayner]. (Jonathan Cape, 1927).

JOURNALS AND PAMPHLETS

THE ANGLO-RUSSIAN HOSPITAL COMMITTEE. *First and Second Prospectuses,* August-September, 1915.

Ibid. *The Work of the Anglo-Russian Hospital;* September 1915 — June 1917. Andrew Fleming and Geoffrey Jefferson.

Ibid. *The Anglo-Russian Hospitals with the Russian Army.* An exhibition at the Grafton Galleries, London; May 1917. Including a brochure of 12 postcards in photogravure showing aspects of the hospital and its field units.

THE BRITISH JOURNAL OF SURGERY, Vol. 5. 1918. *Removal of a Bullet from the Right Lobe of the Cerebellum.* Geoffrey Jefferson, MS, FRCS.

THE BRITISH MEDICAL JOURNAL, 16th October 1917. *Notes from the Anglo-Russian Hospitals.* Sir Herbert F. Waterhouse, FRCS; W. Douglas Harmer, MC, FRCS and Charles J. Marshall, MS, FRCS.

THE BRITISH RED CROSS SOCIETY. *Memories of Russia during the War;* an album of photographs. Mary E. MacDonald.

COUNTRY LIFE, 14th October 1916: Supplement. *The Anglo-Russian Hospital in Petrograd.*

THE NURSING TIMES, 18th September 1915. *The British Hospital, Petrograd.* Janet St. Clair.

THE RED CROSS (Journal of the British Red Cross Society), 15th August 1917. *The Russian Revolution seen from a Hospital Window.* 'V.A.D.'

THE ROYAL COLLEGE OF SURGEONS OF ENGLAND, 1956.
Selected Papers of Sir Geoffrey Jefferson, FRS, MS, FRCS.
Return to Russia.

THE TIMES, 14th September 1915. First list of subscribers to the
A-R H. Appeal Fund.

LETTERS AND DIARIES ETC.

LADY SYBIL GREY. A folio of documents lent by Mr Harry
Middleton. Included are Lady Sybil's accounts of her journey
from Newcastle upon Tyne to Petrograd, the finding of accommodation for the hospital, her visit to the Tsarina at Tsarskoe
Selo, general impressions of war-time life in Petrograd and the
ceremony at the Opera on St. George's Day.

Other pages record the murder of Rasputin and her own
'Diary of Revolution'. In addition there are documents concerning the Revolution which, though of historical interest,
do not bear upon the A-R H. as such.

There are also personal letters to her family and to Lady
Muriel Paget.

W. DOUGLAS HARMER. Fifty-four letters written from Petrograd
and elsewhere, the first dated 12th December (OS 29th
November) 1915; the last dated 21st October 1916. In addition,
a Diary commencing 24th November 1915 and concluding
25th August 1916.

SIR GEOFFREY JEFFERSON. Extracts from 26 letters written
from Petrograd and the Southern Front, the first dated 26th
April 1916, the last dated 28th June 1917. Recorded on tape and
lent by Mr Antony Jefferson, MD, CM, FRCS and Dr Michael
Jefferson, DM, FRCP together with photographs and other
pertinent documents.

LADY MURIEL PAGET. A folio of letters and other documents
lent by Pamela Lady Glenconner. In all there are about 100
letters, written either by Lady Muriel to a wide variety of
recipients or vice versa: of compelling interest. In addition some
documents relating to her subsequent visits to Russia and to her
work for the Distressed British Subjects.

Acknowledgements

In a more gracious age it was customary for an author to end the tail-piece of his book by writing: 'Last but not least I wish to thank my wife for . . .' Many years ago when I was re-editing a standard textbook of Surgery, a task which occupied every spare moment of six years of my professional life, and when we were about to go on a climbing holiday in Cumberland, my wife observed: 'If you take that book with us to the Lakes, I'll throw the damned thing *in* the lake!' In retirement, composition and the necessary research has been easier by far and so first and foremost, I wish not only to acknowledge the support, encouragement, understanding and patience which wives are more or less obliged to give to a scribbling husband but also to record the enthusiam and constructive criticism by which I have been sustained and helped. Were it not that my Essay was dedicated to my father and the Anglo-Russian Hospital, that page would have been inscribed: *For Bridget.*

To my brothers Richard and Christopher I am grateful for permission to make use of my father's letters and diary, and to my sister-in-law Peggy Harmer for valued and constructive criticism.

My debt to the descendants of Lady Muriel Paget and Lady Sybil Middleton can scarcely be computed. The history of the Anglo-Russian Hospitals could have been written of course but without access to the letters which passed between Lady Muriel and Lady Sybil in 1916 and 1917 and which were put at my disposal, it would have been a poor thing indeed. It is with great pleasure therefore that I extend my thanks to Sir John Paget, Lady Chancellor and Pamela Lady Glenconner, the children of Lady Muriel Paget; and to Mr Harry Middleton, Lady Sybil's son, and Mrs David Morse her niece. It is fitting that I should record my particular and personal debt to Pamela Glenconner for keeping me on the straight and narrow path of exactitude by sending me frequent letters recalling incidents in the life of her remarkable mother — many of which unfortunately had no connexion with my tale. She did more: as I submitted my MS for her *nihil obstat* she did not hesitate to criticise the style and format of my writings. To her then, my most profound gratitude.

The list of sources and references which is given in Appendix 6 would have been impossible for me to collect without the help of librarians, archivists, hospital records officers and so on. I therefore express my thanks to the following people and to the Institutions which they represent: Mrs C. F. Fawcett and Miss Margaret Slade (The British Red Cross Society); Mr David Stewart (The Royal Society of Medicine); Mr Eustace Cornelius (The Royal College of Surgeons of England); Mr G. Davenport (The Royal College of Physicians of London); Major-General R. N. Evans, QHP, Commandant and Mrs Sheila McLure, Librarian (The Royal Army Medical College); Miss Marion Tibbetts (The Royal College of Nursing); Mr J. P. Jelley (The General Nursing Council): and to the following hospitals and their officers: Miss M. Culpeck and Miss M. Scholes (The London Hospital); Miss B. Webster (The Royal Free Hospital); Miss E. P. Watt and Miss D. L. Smith (Charing Cross Hospital); and Mr Hugh Anderson (St George's Hospital). In connexion with my search for the 'provenance' of the Matron of the A-R H. I express my thanks to her two nephews Mr J. D. and Mr Alastair Irvine Robertson, who literally came out of the blue to provide me with the necessary information as I was about to conclude my story.

To a number of surgical and medical friends and colleagues I am also most grateful. Dr Michael Jefferson and Mr Antony Jefferson gave me letters and photographs relating to their father; Mr Arthur Makey submitted information about Mr Herbert Waterhouse and Mr Jennings Marshall. Then too, there are Sir Hedley Atkins, Mr Guy Blackburn, Mr Peter Greening and Mr J-C Gazet. Many non-medical persons deserve my thanks as well. My cousin Sir Frederic Harmer and Mr E. L. Colley (of the Ellerman Shipping Lines), were able to identify the courses and fates of some of the ships involved in this account. Mr Frank Bishop of the Shell Transport and Trading Company provided the entirely useless, though quite fascinating, information concerning the value of my mother's shares in his Company. Mr David Buxton (of the Department of Medieval and Later Antiquities of the British Museum) and Mr John Stuart (of Sotheby's) 'researched' St Ouar, the blessed martyr of the BRCS Icon. In other Russian matters I have been privileged to have had the help of Mrs Tamara Talbot-Rice, who explained the intricacies of the Romanov family and gave me many details relating to the years of the Revolution. She was also instrumental in the identification of the author of *The Russian Diary of An Englishman* 'who retired to France following an unfortunate incident in Hyde Park and a short spell at His Majesty's expense'.

My efforts to gain information about the Hospital from the Russian side proved unavailing, although Dr Y. Pavlenko of the USSR Embassy in London and Dr Andrew Rakov, the son of my late surgical friend Professor Alexander Rakov of Leningrad, did their best to help on my behalf. It is sad to have to record that the reply which I received from the Ministry For Public Health in Moscow stated simply that 'after thorough searches which were carried out in different USSR archives the only documents confirming the opening of the Anglo-Russian Hospital on the 1st February 1916 in Petrograd were found. The name of the surgeon V. D. Harmer *(sic)* is in the list of the personnel'.

To the publishers of the following books I acknowledge permission to quote extracts: Methuen & Co *(Lady Muriel)*, Constable & Co *(Nurse at the Russian Front)*, Jonathan Cape *(My Russian Memoirs)*, Faber & Faber *(The British Red Cross in Action)*, Simpkin Marshall & Co *(On The Russian Front)*, and William Heinemann *(The Russian Diary of An Englishman)*. The authors of these books are acknowledged in the text and in the list of references in Appendix 6. As to the first of these — *Lady Muriel* — I hope that I have given adequate expression of my debt to its author, Mr Wilfrid Blunt, in my Prologue.

And last of all an expression of gratitude to friends: to Edward Harber for his superb photograph of my father's bronze uniform badge; to Joanna White for her elegant map of the Eastern Front; to Richard Garnett of Macmillans but above all to Elwyn Owen-Jones of the Chichester Press who guided me through the devious paths of printing and publishing; and to two others in particular who I am bold enough to describe (in Lady Sybil's phraseology of course) as my personal slaves — Sara James and Sandra Hill. It was they who did the hard work of typing the manuscript, not once but many a time on account of my persistent alterations.

I have indeed been fortunate in the enthusiastic support which I have been given by everyone concerned in my attempt to put on record the history of a most noble enterprise. As far as I can say, the story of the Anglo-Russian Hospital has not been told before. Perhaps this Essay may stimulate someone one day to do it better.